Psychoanalytically Informed Play Therapy

Psychoanalytically Informed Play Therapy: Fantasy-Exposure Life-Narrative Therapy is a structured manual for the execution of FELT, an integrative play therapy that marries the analytic, relational, and psychodynamic aspects of traditional Play Therapy with the scientific rigor and replicability standards of clinical empiricism.

Jason Steadman's FELT model creates a structured, empirically derived means of monitoring children's play using psychoanalytic methods. Steadman's method proposes the usage of story stems to structure play to address critical needs in children's psychological development. In FELT, Steadman teaches readers how to identify problematic play themes and how to respond therapeutically to drive play and general child development toward healthy directions. Steadman uses anxiety as the primary example of psychological distress for FELT, but also shows how the method can be applied to many other pathologies, such as depression and trauma. Steadman explains 11 core FELT themes, which are then further condensed to three major clinical targets identified in the play of clinically anxious children. Each of these is described in detail in the book and therapists are shown not only how to reliably identify themes, but how to focus their interventions to move children toward major play-based targets. Integrating psychoanalytic theory with an emphasis on Object Relations, Steadman's FELT program highlights the importance of the self in healthy child development and how play-based psychotherapy can be used to help children build stronger, healthier selves that can face a wide variety of psychological issues across their lifespan.

Including comprehensive theoretical underpinnings and thorough clinical examples of FELT at work, this volume will allow therapists, clinicians, and mental health workers to understand childhood play in an empirically based manner and show them how to integrate the key tenets of FELT into their own work to better aid children experiencing anxiety and other mental health concerns.

Dr. Jason L. Steadman received his doctorate in clinical psychology from Baylor University in 2014. He is a board-certified clinical child psychologist currently working in full-time practice in Chattanooga, Tennessee.

Psychoanalytically Informed Play Therapy

Fantasy-Exposure Life-Narrative Therapy

Jason L. Steadman

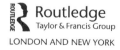

Routledge
Taylor & Francis Group

LONDON AND NEW YORK

Designed cover image: © Getty

First published 2024
by Routledge
4 Park Square, Milton Park, Abingdon, Oxon OX14 4RN

and by Routledge
605 Third Avenue, New York, NY 10158

Routledge is an imprint of the Taylor & Francis Group, an informa business

© 2024 Jason L. Steadman

British Library Cataloguing-in-Publication Data
A catalogue record for this book is available from the British Library

ISBN: 978-1-032-69316-3 (hbk)
ISBN: 978-1-032-64656-5 (pbk)
ISBN: 978-1-032-69318-7 (ebk)

DOI: 10.4324/9781032693187

Typeset in Times New Roman
by Taylor & Francis Books

Access the Support Material: www.routledge.com/9781032693163

Special thanks to Helen Benedict and Elizabeth Coe

For Aiyana and Pato

Contents

List of illustrations   xiii

PART I
Background, theory, and conceptualization   I

1 An introduction to play and storytelling   3

   Defining therapeutic play 6
   Storytelling 7
   Overview of the rest of the book 9

2 Fantasy-Exposure Life-Narrative Therapy: Its development and
   an overview of the format   11

   The core tenets of Play Therapy 12
   FELT treatment fidelity checklist 15
   The FELT format – play analysis through story stems 15
      A preface about coding 16
      Initial response 18
      Final content 19
      Deus ex machina resolution 21
      Emotional shift 23
      Incongruent affect 24
      Reactions to inescapable fear/anxiety 27
      Danger 28
      Neediness 29
      Labeling of emotions and symptoms 31
      Self-representations 31
      "Other" representations 33
      The prime maladaptive themes 34

FELT designed as a treatment for anxiety 36

3   Object-relations theory in child development and in childhood
play   39

The Self 39
    Postmodern views of the Self 42
    Self-representations and traits: how we use words to define
    the Self 43
*Therapeutic goals that derive from vulnerabilities of the Self
across childhood 51*
    Goals for Self-development in very early childhood (ages 2–
    4) 51
    Goals for Self-development in early to middle childhood
    (ages 5–7) 53
    Goals for Self-development in middle to late childhood
    (ages 8–11) 54
Objects 55
    Internal representations of Objects 56
The "in-between" – the relationship between Self and Objects 68
The accuracy of internal representations 71
*Real versus imagined relationships and their impact on Object-
relations 72*

4   Mechanisms of change in psychotherapy   76

Expression, catharsis, and labeling of feelings 76
Corrective emotional experience 76
Insight, re-experiencing, and working through 77
    Analgesia/comfort needs 77
    Need for power: *dunamis* and *exousia* needs 79
    Superego needs 79
    Need for love 80
    Need for Objects 81
    Popularity needs 82
    Integration needs 83
    Other core psychoanalytic ideas influencing how change
    occurs in psychotherapy 85
    Insight, re-experiencing, and working through: summary 88
Problem-solving techniques and coping strategies 88

Object-relations, internal representations, and interpersonal development 89
Overlapping mechanisms in integrative therapy 90

5 Core principles of effective therapy: The ACER characteristics   92

Attunement 92
Concern 94
Expertise 94
Responsivity 95
Summary 96

6 FELT etiological model of anxiety   98

The FELT anxiety model 98
Propagating factors 100
     Genetic factors 100
     Psychodynamic factors 101
     Environmental/cultural/learned factors 103
Manifest factors 107
     Biological dysfunction 108
     Negative affect 108
Temporal factors 111
What does all this mean for FELT? 116

7 Pharmacology and biological factors of childhood anxiety   122

Pharmacological approaches to anxiety treatment 122
     What are the clinical targets of medications used to treat
     anxiety? 123
     Physiological arousal and distress in anxious humans 127
*Behavioral and psychotherapeutic means to match biological
   needs 131*
     Fulfillment 131
     Sedation/de-arousal 131
     Behavioral improvement of serotonin function 133
Conclusion: key points from Part I of this book 134

PART II
Session guides and story stem creation   137

8 The FELT treatment outlined by session   139

Before starting FELT – materials needed 139
Guidelines for all sessions 139
Session 1 144
    Purpose 144
    Goals 144
    Methods 144
    Activity 1: Getting to know each other 145
    Activity 2: Introduction to therapy 147
    Activity 3: A happy time 148
Session 2 – "Feelings are important" 150
    Purpose 150
    Goals 150
    Activity 1: A positive feeling 150
    Activity 2: Worry time 151
    Activity 3: Client-specific anxiety 155
    Closing the session 157
Session 3 – Somatic anxiety 158
    Purpose 158
    Goals 158
    Activity 1: Signs of worry 158
    [OPTIONAL] Activity 2: Child-specific anxiety story 162
    Closing remarks 162
In between sessions 3 and 4 162
Session 4 163
    Purpose 163
    Goals 163
    Activity 1: Talking about the parent session 164
    Activity 2: Physiological reactivity 164
    Activity 3: Relaxing 167
    Activity 4: Progressive muscle relaxation story 170
    Activity 5: Parents 171
    Worrying William/Wendy story stems 172
In between sessions 4 and 5 173
    Case conceptualization, with an example 173
Session 5 – Self-talk and maladaptive thought patterns 178
    Purpose 178

Goals 178
Activity 1: Physiology and relaxation review 178
Activity 2: Vet visit 178
Activity 3: Vet visit, reversed roles 180
Session 6 183
Purpose 183
Goals 183
Activity 1: Physiology and relaxation 184
Activity 2: Anxious thoughts review 184
Activity 3: Assessment and reward 185
Session 7 190
Purpose 190
Goals 190
Activity 1: Physiology and relaxation 190
Activity 2: Anxious thoughts 190
Activity 3: Self-efficacy review 192
Sessions 8–12+ 192
Goals 193
Story stems 194

9 Parent component 199

*Parent-only session (in development studies, this came after
session 3 with child) 199*
Purpose 199
Goals and tasks 200
Parents' involvement in session 4 with child and afterward 202
Preventing premature termination 203

10 Termination 206

Termination stems 207
A gorilla is released back into the wild 207
A hospitalized child is released from hospital 209
Other termination stories 209
Termination session 209
Termination activities 210
Sample termination book 211

11 Creating your own story stems 219

What makes a story therapeutic? 219

Choosing a tension point 221
  Example 1: Jane creates a story to address *dunamis* fear 223
  Example 2: Chris addresses superego needs 225
  Multilayered stories 227
  Example 3: Brett creates a story to simultaneously address
    needs for *exousia* and for love 227
A template for story creation 230

12 Future directions   233

  Adapting for depressive disorders 233

  Index   241

Illustrations

Figures

6.1	FELT etiological model of anxiety	99
8.1	A basic set-up of the child–therapist play interview. Photo by author.	149
8.2	Emotions circumplex: example	150
8.3	Robbers breaking in upstairs during the Robber stem. In this example, the child is running outside to get help from her mother, who is outside working in the garden. Photo by author.	160
8.4	This image shows a variation on activity 5.3. In this case, rather than birds, the vet visits with two giraffes and a gazelle. Photo by author.	181
8.5	A basic set-up for the Music concert stem, close up, no audience. Photo by author.	191
10.1	Gorillas, after temporarily residing at the zoo, are preparing to be released back into the wild. In this image, some of the zoo staff slept on top of the enclosure to be near to the gorillas (an addition suggested by the child who played this scene). Photo by author.	208

Tables

2.1	The FELT play themes	17
3.1	Norms and abnormalities of Self-development from ages 2 to 11	52
8.1	List of items/toys needed for FELT	140
8.2	Interoceptive exposure activities for children and anxiety symptoms each is designed to mimic	165
10.1	Guide/Example for termination book	212

Part I

Background, theory, and conceptualization

Chapter 1

An introduction to play and storytelling

Play is the quintessential childhood experience. Left to their own devices, children will find ways to play during any circumstance. Play is the language through which children communicate with others about the world, and importantly, about what they think about the world. Play is also incredibly important for child development. It is how children build relationships and skills that will serve them throughout their lives, even into adulthood.

Play begins at a very young age, even during the first month of life. Healthy, neurotypical infants are biologically rooted to make eye contact with their caregivers. They also recognize their parent's (parents') voice(s), showing a differential response to familiar voices than unfamiliar voices. These sensory reactions – eye contact and voice recognition – are the earliest signs of social contact and, also, the earliest signs of the capacity for play. Instinctively, adults play with these sensory experiences through games of peek-a-boo, by using "baby talk" to make their voice more interesting, and by smiling frequently at the baby. Similarly, we dance with our babies, by wiggling their little arms and legs, giving them important exercise and stimulation, or by rocking them to sleep while singing a lullaby, teaching them early that play can be sometimes stimulating and sometimes relaxing, depending on what you're doing. Play continues to develop in increasingly interesting ways throughout a child's life, varying with their cognitive, emotional, and overall psychological development.

Though not all definitions of play are equal in what they consider play and what they do not, there are a few core features of play that will form the definition I use in this book. First, play is fun. Play can include any activity that includes pleasure among its primary purposes. However, although play is enjoyable, it need not always be *fully* enjoyable to count as play. Anyone who has ever played anything knows that play can stimulate a wide variety of feelings, both pleasurable and less-pleasurable feelings. When I was a kid, I was hurt by and did hurt others through play. I also hurt myself on occasion. In fact, play is probably the leading cause of accidental childhood injury.[1] According to a 2016 publication by the US Consumer Product Safety Commission (CPSC, 2016), during 2012–2014, US emergency departments treated

DOI: 10.4324/9781032693187-2

247,075 each year for playground-related injuries. So, sometimes play hurts, physically. Play can hurt emotionally too. During play, people commonly experience frustration, rage, sadness, grief, and an array of other negative emotions. So, play doesn't have to *always* be fun to count as play. Nevertheless, a key definitive component of play is that it is at least partially fun, or intended to be fun.

Another important feature of the definition of play is that play is metaphor. In other words, many actions carried out through play are not intended to be interpreted literally. However, playful actions often carry a metaphorical message. Pretend (fantasy) play is the most obvious form of playful metaphor. Even though children, especially young children, seem at times to get so engaged in fantasy that they seem to believe what they're playing is real, when pressed (in the right way), almost all children can tell a difference between fantasy and reality. They understand, intuitively, that they are "just playing," and not actually carrying out a complex war among their action figures or baking a real cake when using their Easy-Bake Oven. Still, the metaphor of play carries important messages that are essential to a child's development. It is through metaphor that children can safely explore vital life skills within the safety of the play environment. They can make mistakes; they can explore death; they can show aggression; they can play "mommy," all without worrying about actually killing someone or maintaining the real responsibilities of parenthood.

Third, in addition to being fun and involving metaphor, for many, play counts as anything that is not "work." Although the distinction is not always exact – some work can feel like play and some play can feel like work – many people define "play time" as any time that is free of the responsibilities and expectations of work. This brings us to another core definition of play used in this book: relative to work, *play is often automatic and unfiltered.* When we work, humans usually put effort into making sure that work fits a certain "prototype" – matching whatever standard the work expects from us. Play, on the other hand, has no prototype. Play can be and become anything. It is not limited by expectations, and, as a result, when humans play, we do not have to effortfully control every aspect of the play to fit into a certain mold. Sometimes, work and play intermingle. It is possible for some aspects of our work to have playful components, and it is possible for play to employ at least a small amount of work. Professional athletes are good examples of this. They play a game for a living, but they are also under (sometimes immense) pressure to produce a certain result every time they play (work). The same could be argued for professional musicians, or builders, or teachers, or play therapists, or any profession that has managed the dream of turning a playful activity into a career. All such professionals straddle the line between work and play, and, if we're not careful, the "work" parts of such jobs overtake the "play," and vice versa. When we're adults, the "work" part is more likely to take precedence, because adults are more able to put our responsibilities ahead of our sense of fun, sometimes to our own detriment. In children, on the other hand, the "play" part is more likely to take precedence. In most tasks that involve both play and work, children are more likely to automatically revert toward the play, in which they simply bask in the enjoyment of unfiltered freedom.

Unfortunately, we adults often spend quite a lot of time hammering that tendency to play out of children, and we've been doing it at increasingly high rates over the last several decades. From 1981 to 1997, children's playtime decreased by 25%, and children aged 3–11 years had a decrease of 12 hours per week of free time (Sandberg & Hofferth, 2001). Furthermore, increases in academic pressures are notable in numerous educational policy changes. Recent data, in fact, show that 30% of US Kindergarten children do not have (outdoor) recess (Murray et al., 2013). Among my own clients, across more than 20 different elementary schools in three different states, I cannot think of a single one who feels satisfied by the amount of recess/play they get every day. These trends have happened because we've grown increasingly focused, in our society, on preparing children's brains to reach adulthood earlier. We want them to be more like us, able to prioritize work over play as soon as they hit school. Sure, at some point it is wise to teach children to be able to "suck it up" and "get a job done," even if they don't really feel like it and even if the job isn't totally "fun," because that is a very important skill for success in adulthood. Still, we must be careful not to suck all the fun out of childhood as we strive to teach them the responsibilities of adulthood. This principle applies to psychotherapy too. To best connect with children, psychotherapy should be at least minimally playful.

Another consequence of adulthood is that we often forget how to play. For many of us, work consumes a lot of energy, and by the time we finally have time to play, we don't really have the energy for it. Many adults, then, end up "stuck" in a continuous, repetitive rut of always doing what we have to do, and we don't take time to enjoy the automaticity and freedom of play. Furthermore, when many adults play, we put constraints on the play. Adults don't mean to do this. It comes, simply, from, a lifetime of being taught to do things a certain way. As a result, many adults tend to judge our own and others' play in ways that children do not. Adults set expectations for what play "should" look like, and we judge or correct the play if it does not meet those expectations. These judgments have the capacity to push out the characteristics that make play what it is – the fun, the metaphor, the automaticity – and instead change it into work – making it serious, unimaginative, and purposeful. Thus, one of the greatest things we can do as adults who work with children is to let them teach us how to play again – to have fun, to imagine, and to be free.

At the same time, we adults can use our maturity and wisdom to respond to and guide children's play in meaningful ways. All children will, eventually, through play express chaos. They will hit a wall where they do not know how to resolve conflict that has arisen in play, and they will inevitably need the guidance of an experienced, wise mentor to promote resolution of this conflict. In fact, this feature is the fourth key component of our definition of play used here – play promotes and allows skill building through scaffolding and interpersonal exchange. It is through social play that children build important skills in learning how to manage social exchanges throughout their lives, but without interference from others, most play in early childhood is prone to social conflict. In other words, toddlers playing together will eventually fight, and they rely on adults or other children to help resolve the fights that occur in play. Thus, play allows a safe exchange for social skills in a relatively low-risk environment.

Given play is a realm for the practice of social skills, play is often an intensely interpersonal exchange. Play doesn't just allow for social skills practice, it also allows participants to engage in reciprocal interactions that communicate emotional, cognitive, and general psychological states. Thus, interpersonal play does more than build social skills, it allows children (and adults too) to express their internal selves to another person. In reciprocal exchange of these internal states, a process we'll call *attunement*, which will be defined later in this book, important therapeutic processes occur which allow the possibility for these internal states to resolve in natural, healthy ways. Put more simply, because play involves the communication of meaningful thoughts, feelings, and behaviors between players, play opens a world of internal psychology that often does not arise naturally in other contexts. By listening to the internal psychology of players, we professionals can better understand how children think and feel about their world, which we can then guide, as needed, toward healthier outcomes.

In summary, then, play is defined in this book to contain several important features: 1) play is (at least partially) fun, 2) play uses metaphor, 3) play is relatively unfiltered, 4) play promotes skill building, and 5) the metaphor of childhood play carries messages that demand an interpersonal response from another.

Defining therapeutic play

The preceding section defined play in general, but it is also important to distinguish that not all play is "created equally," so to speak. Some play may have more of the five above characteristics than other types, and some play, even with the above characteristics, can still be destructive to kids, rather than therapeutic. Some play, such as rules-based play or "game" play (e.g., sports, a game of chess, board games, etc.), may not contain much metaphor and may not be very "free" or unfiltered. Some kids (e.g., kids on the autism spectrum or other rigid thinkers) can find unfiltered (unstructured) play to be anxiety-provoking. For them, then, "free-play" is decidedly not fun. In both examples, play is arguably still happening on some levels, but not on others, and that play can still be considered therapeutic, even if it doesn't contain all five of the features of play defined in this chapter.

Another key distinction is the point at which play becomes "therapeutic." For the purposes of this book, therapeutic play is defined as any type of playful activity that results in meaningful, *healthy* change in at least one of the players. Of course, this feature begs the question: What defines "healthy" change? Healthy change is defined by the empirically supported personality characteristics of healthy children. These characteristics are further defined in later chapters on child development and "normal" childhood play. Still, play becomes therapeutic when it facilitates a child's development toward a healthy norm. We also define "healthy" play, in part, by studying the play of "unhealthy" children and comparing that to the play of healthy children. Features that are consistently present in the play of "unhealthy" children, but not in "healthy" children, then, could be used to define "unhealthy" play. Play analysis, including ways to differentiate "healthy" from "unhealthy" play, is outlined in depth in Chapter 2 of this book.

The remaining focus of this book, interwoven throughout and across each chapter, guides therapists and other interested professionals who work with children in *how* to design and structure interventions that lead children toward healthy play. The program outlined herein utilizes a combination of directive and non-directive play-based approaches to facilitate children's movement toward healthy play. The techniques are most appropriate for child therapists with specific, prerequisite mental health training. However, some of the techniques can also be used by parents, teachers, doctors, and anyone else who is given the responsibility of raising mentally healthy children.

Storytelling

FELT integrates narrative storytelling techniques to help facilitate therapeutic play. In fact, the primary therapeutic component of FELT is in the exploration and manipulation of personal narratives toward healthy directions, not in the play itself. Play is the mechanism through which storytelling and narrative work is executed, but the therapeutic content is found in the narrative, not in the play itself. So, it is absolutely essential that professionals who use FELT understand and effectively use storytelling in their work.

To be effective, though, professionals do *not* need to be, themselves, master storytellers. My first faculty position was at East Tennessee State University (ETSU), and at my new-faculty orientation, I won two VIP tickets to the National Storytelling Festival, held annually in Jonesborough, TN, about 20 minutes from ETSU. I was told this was an excellent prize, but having never heard of this festival before, I didn't really understand what I had won. I did attend though, and it was there that I first learned what truly masterful storytelling looked (and sounded) like. Well, I can tell you, I created FELT – a storytelling-focused psychotherapy – and I am nothing like those storytellers. You do not have to be, either.

Children tend to be more easily pleased by stories than adults. Children will not judge you for the "logic," or the concision, or for the performance of stories you tell in therapy. So, you do not have to worry about "putting on a show," as part of your therapeutic storytelling in FELT. Furthermore, stories in FELT are told collaboratively with children. Narratives created in FELT are not performances where the storyteller knows the beginning, middle, and end of the story from the start. Rather, they are working narratives that grow and change according to the needs of the child in session. So, the storytelling tasks of FELT are less about telling stories, but, rather, more about conducting effective psychotherapy through stories, and, more specifically, through story stems. More information on this process is outlined in subsequent chapters, where essential components of therapeutic stories are outlined in detail. Here, I will focus on a basic overview.

Stories connect best with audiences when they are familiar. So, a major part of narrative therapy with children is in first learning what is familiar to them. To tell stories with children, you should first know children in general, but you should also know your specific audience – the child in front of you. At the storytelling festival I mentioned above, the storytellers told stories in the Appalachian tradition, because that was their audience (and possibly because the festival organizers recruited such storytellers, because they knew the audience would be mostly Appalachian folk). Had the conference been held in a more urban area, I suspect the stories would have had a more urban feel. Or, if the audience were predominantly Chinese-Americans, the stories would have had a Chinese influence. The point is that in order to tell an engaging story to your audience, you must know your audience. This is one reason that early sessions in FELT are structured to be "learning" sessions – to get to know the child in front of you. This is also why early sessions consist of generalized story stems, rather than targeted ones. The generalized stems were designed to be relevant to a general audience of anxious children, and they use themes that are familiar to most children. It is only later in FELT, after therapists have gotten to know their specific clients better, that targeted story stems are introduced and used more readily. It can be said, then, that over time, FELT therapists increase the familiarity of the stories to each specific child receiving FELT. Using familiarity to create targeted stories is outlined in more detail in Chapter 11.

Familiarity not only increases engagement, but it is also a key component of what makes a story more likely to be therapeutic. Therapeutic stories are ones that connect relevantly to important aspects of a person's life and then change (for the better) our perspectives about those particular aspects. Therapeutic storytelling has been around since the beginning of time, as evidenced by the story structures of ancient cave paintings, which often appear to depict real-life events. Presumably, our ancestors used stories of real-life events to communicate their personal history and their struggles to find food and provide safety and security for their families and tribes. These stories likely helped teach children about adult life and about the responsibilities of family and tribal leadership. They captured what was familiar to children – their daily lives – and created narratives around those events to teach important lessons. Therapeutic stories today are no different. So, in order to be truly therapeutic, stories must connect to the real-life experiences of the audience, such that, through the lens of the story, the audience now gains a different (even if only by a tiny increment) outlook on the events contained in the story.

Of course, familiarity does not mean that stories must be fully congruent with the real-life experiences of children. The real-life experiences of clinically anxious children are characterized by problematic responses to anxious stimuli. These problematic responses do not need to be recreated and then left unresolved in psychotherapy. In fact, such a story would probably serve to exacerbate anxiety, rather than ameliorate it. Rather, stories should deviate away from problematic responding and instead toward healthy exemplars. By creating and telling stories that show healthy responding, children learn then to generalize such healthy exemplars to the real world, and they can then use those same positive coping skills outside of therapy. So, a therapist's task is to create enough familiarity such that children are engaged and able to connect stories to their actual experiences, while simultaneously generating new, unique experiences through stories that children can then take into their real lives.

Overview of the rest of the book

In subsequent chapters, I will provide a comprehensive overview of the FELT program, which will include theoretical underpinnings essential to FELT's reliable implementation, as well as concrete examples of what activities are actually performed within FELT sessions. Chapter 2 provides an overview of FELT's format, starting from its initial development and then moving into detailed coverage of play and narrative analysis. After reading Chapter 2, therapists should have a heightened awareness of structured, analytic coding systems and how these are used to understand childhood play in an empirically based manner. FELT is heavily influenced by Object-relations theory, and the psychotherapeutic relationship in FELT is often described and conceptualized in Object-relational terms. Chapter 3 is dedicated to an extensive overview of Object-relations theory as it plays out in child development and in FELT. Chapter 4 further explores mechanisms of change in psychotherapy. FELT is a theoretically integrative approach to psychotherapy. Consequently, in order to execute FELT well, it helps for therapists to have a strong working knowledge of how change occurs across multiple approaches and theoretical orientations, so that they may then use techniques taken from each orientation effectively in sessions. In Chapter 5, I then take the lessons learned from various mechanisms of change to propose a comprehensive model of therapist characteristics necessary to facilitate change. This model, called the ACER model, describes how therapists must be attuned, concerned, experts, who are responsive to the needs and personal goals of their clients.

Chapter 6 describes a complex etiological model for childhood anxiety that guides therapists in identifying therapeutic targets for intervention. The FELT etiological model is designed to be a therapist's model, rather than a scientific model. In other words, although the model does derive from empirically supported resources, the focus of the FELT etiological model is not in presenting another testable theory about how anxiety develops. Plenty of those already exist. Rather, the focus of the FELT etiological model is to present a means through which therapists can identify how to treat anxiety using the multiple theoretical approaches outlined in Chapter 4. It concretizes several factors essential to managing childhood anxiety. It is also a multi-theoretical model. Readers will recognize most heavily components from psychodynamic theory and cognitive behavioral theory. Chapter 7 also provides coverage over biological factors associated with anxiety and how these are treated through pharmacotherapy and through behavioral principles. After reading Chapters 6 and 7, therapists should be armed with an array of advanced ideas to guide how they choose to intervene in childhood anxiety.

Part II of this book, Session Guides and Story Stem Creation, presents the actual session content of FELT. Before attempting to implement FELT with actual clients, therapists should read Part II in its entirety. Chapter 8 includes session-by-session outlines with goals and suggested activities for each session. Chapter 9 separately, and briefly, outlines the parent component of FELT. Chapter 10 outlines procedures for the planned conclusion of therapy, and Chapter 11 provides instructions and guidance for therapists to create their own, targeted story stems in therapy.

The book concludes with a "Future directions" chapter in Chapter 12, where I briefly comment about plans to adapt FELT for use with disorders other than anxiety.

Note

1 Because of the way physicians record injuries, there are no good statistical studies that clearly show the rates of all injury as a result of play. Instead, injuries are usually recorded as being due to a fall or being struck by an object or due to a burn, without always specifying if the injury occurred during a type of play.

REFERENCES

Consumer Product Safety Commission (CPSC). (2016). Injuries and investigated deaths associated with playground equipment, 2009–2014. Bethesda, MD: U.S. Consumer Product Safety Commission. https://www.cpsc.gov/s3fs-public/Injuries%20and%20Investigated%20Deaths%20Associated%20with%20Playground%20Equipment%202009%20to%202014_1.pdf.

Murray, R., Ramstetter, C., Council on School Health, & American Academy of Pediatrics. (2013). The crucial role of recess in school. *Pediatrics*, 131(1), 183–188.

Sandberg, J. F., & Hofferth, S. L. (2001). Changes in children's time with parents: United States, 1981–1997. *Demography*, 38(3), 423–436.

Chapter 2

Fantasy-Exposure Life-Narrative Therapy

Its development and an overview of the format

Fantasy-Exposure Life-Narrative Therapy (FELT) came to life around mid-2011, when I was a graduate student at Baylor University and began planning my dissertation. As a student, I became interested in bolstering the empirical basis for Play Therapy as a discipline, which has a long, fruitful clinical history but which, regrettably, continues to suffer from criticisms by empiricists that it lacks support, relative to Cognitive Behavioral Therapy (CBT), in particular, for it being an effective approach with most childhood conditions. Critics, for the most part, argue that Play Therapy as a whole is not very effective at all, or, at least, that there is relatively limited rigorous empirical evidence supporting Play Therapy (Higa-McMillan et al., 2016; Bratton et al., 2005; Phillips, 2010). Further, they argue that when it is effective, it is due not to the play components of the model, but to the execution of other, better-established interventions that just happen to come about during play. FELT, then, was designed mainly as an attempt to bridge the gap between Play Therapy purists – those who truly believe in the natural, direct, healing powers of play – and Play Therapy critics – those who see play as a mere mode of carrying out other empirically supported interventions, such as CBT.

FELT was written with these goals specifically in mind. I wanted to maintain fidelity to the traditions of Play Therapy purists while also building a program that could be studied with the same empirical rigor as more structured programs common to CBT. To do so, I kept several features in mind during development.

Features of Play Therapy:

- Analysis of play themes
- Focus on the impact of the therapeutic relationship
- Using psychodynamic theories to explain and understand the development of pathology
- Play itself as the primary tool for directing therapeutic change
- Focus on play, and changes in the play itself, as a primary marker of healthy change

DOI: 10.4324/9781032693187-3

Features of empirically supported treatments:

• Reproducible in research
• Clearly delineated and potentially observable mechanism of change
• Contains clear goals and guidelines to be followed by therapists

This chapter covers the core theories that influenced and shaped the development of FELT from both a clinical and an empirical perspective.

The core tenets of Play Therapy

In the section below, I'll provide a very cursory review of some of Play Therapy history and from where some of the classic core tenets of Play Therapy originally derived. Readers should know that this section is not intended to cover the extreme richness and depth that exists in Play Therapy theory and practice. Rather, I will limit myself to brief, historical references, mainly to set a stage/structure for understanding core features of FELT.

Play Therapy was developed originally out of the theories of Melanie Klein, Anna Freud, Margaret Lowenfield, and Virginia Axline. Klein is best known as a child psychoanalyst, and she believed strongly in psychoanalytic play technique and play analysis. It is from her pioneering work, influenced by Sigmund Freud's psychoanalytic techniques, that analysis of childhood play became mainstream. Klein was an active analyst, interpreting children's play from the onset of therapy and believing that these interpretations directly affected (healed) childhood psychopathology. Klein was also a pioneer of Object-relations theory, which is explored in depth in Chapter 3.

Anna Freud (Sigmund's daughter) took a similar approach to her father and to Klein, but she wrote more extensively about some of the technical limitations of analysis with children, due to their underdeveloped superegos and limited verbal skills. As a result, Freud generally offered fewer interpretations than Klein, but focused instead on the therapeutic relationship with the child.

Lowenfield is best known for creating the now widely used methods of sand trays and water trays, along with miniatures, to create "worlds" in play. Central to modern Play Therapy training, "world building" with miniatures is a foundation of Play Therapy, and many modern therapists write extensively about the unique features that sand and water play bring to therapy (see O'Connor, Schaefer, & Braverman, 2016). Without Lowenfield's foundation, though, the use of miniatures and world-building in Play Therapy today may never have grown to its current status.

Virginia Axline, though her work came later than Klein, Freud, and Lowenfield, is often credited as the "mother of play therapy" (Johnson, 2016, p. 22). Her groundbreaking books *Play Therapy: The Inner Dynamics of Childhood* (1947) and *Dibs in Search of Self* (1964) are among the most famous in all of Play Therapy literature, the former a more textbook-like overview of Axline's Play Therapy technique, and the latter an engaging case study that reads like a novel. Personally, I recommend *Dibs* to all of my students of Play Therapy, if for nothing else than just that it is a darned good book that gives readers tremendous hope about the healing powers of play. Axlinean technique is best described as child-centered Play Therapy. Axline herself was an acolyte of Carl Rogers, having studied directly under him, and his influence on her work is clear, with both sharing ideas about the necessary components of therapy that allow a client to "self-heal." For Axline, the necessary components of Play Therapy – her "eight basic principles" (Axline, 1974) – included 1) warmth (a friendly relationship); 2) acceptance; 3) permissiveness (for the child to freely express the Self); 4) therapist recognition and reflection of expressed feelings, communicated back to the child in order to give insight; 5) respect for autonomy (it is the child's responsibility to change); 6) non-directiveness ("the child leads the way; the therapist follows") (p. 73); 7) patience (the therapist does not try to hurry therapy); and 8) structuring (which in this case meant setting enough limits to establish with the child the nature and purpose of therapy).

As a conscious effort to maintain some of the "purity" of Play Therapy models, FELT follows the traditions established by the founders of Play Therapy. FELT includes play analysis, as pioneered by Klein, but with careful recognition that not all children respond to analysis in the same way, and they certainly respond differently than adults (a lesson from Freud). Though FELT does not require the use of sand or water play, FELT does assume play is a collaborative creation of "worlds," for which Lowenfield must be given credit. Finally, FELT includes a staunch focus on necessary characteristics of the therapist which help facilitate therapeutic growth in children.

Many of these components of Play Therapy, and how they integrate into FELT, are outlined in later chapters of this book (specifically, Chapter 3 on Object-relations theory; Chapter 4 on mechanisms of change in psychotherapy; Chapter 5 on interpersonal features of effective therapy; and Chapter 6 on case conceptualization). In the current chapter, I focus on play analysis. More precisely, I present an evidence-based, structured form of play analysis that can be learned and implemented by any therapist. The analytic approach used in FELT is borrowed from research-based paradigms that have been in use for decades (since at least the early 1990s), but, to my knowledge, FELT is the first to apply the designs used in analytic research to a manualized, therapeutic paradigm. Thus, FELT is meant not just to be a presentation of another model of Play Therapy; it is also a presentation of a means to design analytic play therapies to withstand rigorous research analyses.

Importantly, although FELT is a play therapy, for professionals who are learning/using FELT, the play is work. This goes back to some of the distinctions defining play outlined in Chapter 1, perhaps most importantly the component of play that makes it unfiltered and automatic. From the therapist's perspective, FELT requires constant work – work before the session to plan and prepare, work during the session to interpret play reactions and respond accordingly, and work in between sessions to conceptualize the client and adapt the FELT plan to fit the individual conceptualization. Although it may appear to an outside onlooker that FELT therapists are only "playing" in therapy, the therapist is working diligently and assiduously throughout to apply therapeutic principles to the play. Still, because FELT can look, at times, to observers (especially to parents) like undirected, random play, it is *essential* for therapists to communicate openly with others about the FELT therapeutic model and the mechanisms through which FELT accomplishes therapeutic change in children. For this reason, understanding the core principles of Play Therapy (proper) and of evidence-based psychotherapy in general are essential for competent practice of FELT. Communicating therapeutic mechanisms with others not only provides reassurances to parents about what is happening in individual sessions, it also provides parents with essential learning necessary for them to replicate therapeutic play at home.

FELT was also designed as a contextual psychotherapy. Many manualized approaches to therapy are disease/disorder specific. They are "prescribed" to treat conditions and are studied under ideal conditions with patients who meet specific inclusion and exclusion criteria. Although the studies that support FELT do use a rigorous design, targeting specific populations (i.e., children with anxiety disorders) and using methodologies typical of "laboratory-based" intervention research (see Steadman, 2016), the manual itself is written to be adapted to each individual client. Thus, FELT is intended to be a training program for general, evidence-based Play Therapy skills. In studies so far, these skills have been practiced and evaluated primarily with anxious preschool and elementary-aged children, but the skills can also apply to a wide array of childhood-presenting complaints, and it is my sincere hope that future studies will expand on FELT skills to investigate their utility with other childhood psychiatric conditions/complaints. These ideas are discussed further in the final section of this chapter and again in the conclusion of the book (Chapter 12).

Because FELT is contextual, it invokes a mixture of generalized and client-specific interventions over the course of a therapeutic trial. There are some generalized interventions that are used with every client to whom FELT is applied, while client-specific interventions rely on general FELT principles to design and implement interventions that address core issues presented by each individual child (and/or their parents). The manual does include session-by-session prompts/goals, and the front half of the entire program (the first several sessions) is much heavier on generalized approaches, while the latter half gets more client specific, as the therapist gets to know the child better over time. However, fidelity tracking (how well a therapist does at following FELT principles) does not rely on whether or not a therapist adheres to session-by-session outlines. Rather, fidelity relies completely on adherence to the general principles of FELT outlined throughout this book. This format of fidelity monitoring emphasizes the fact that the FELT paradigm focuses more heavily on effective therapeutic *techniques* than it does on the execution of specific interventions or coping outcomes during FELT. A copy of the FELT fidelity checklist used in FELT studies is included below. This checklist is not meant for general use. Instead, it is meant as a tool for a FELT trainer/supervisor to monitor how well a therapist-in-training is using FELT according to protocol. It is included here merely as an example of what I consider to be most essential to FELT training and FELT fidelity. The checklist uses rather generic, vague terminology (e.g., the therapist is attuned…), and the details of these terms and what they really mean in the FELT model will emerge throughout this manual. As you read through this manual, you are encouraged to revisit this fidelity checklist and ponder what kinds of things a FELT trainer would look for in sessions as evidence that these skills were executed in session.

FELT treatment fidelity checklist

Please rate the therapist along the following dimensions. For definitions of terms, see the treatment manual.

  0 = never, 1 = rarely, 2 = sometimes, 3 = often, 4 = almost always, DK = don't know

  1   The therapy is play-based.0 1 2 3 4 DK
  2   The play is characterized by metaphor and symbolism.0 1 2 3 4 DK
  3   The therapist demonstrates clear evidence they have analyzed the child's play for themes. 0 1 2 3 4 DK
  4   The therapist uses themes to inform play-based responses.0 1 2 3 4 DK
  5   The therapist is attuned to the child.0 1 2 3 4 DK
  6   The therapist displays concern for the child.0 1 2 3 4 DK
  7   The therapist intervenes therapeutically when opportunities arise. 0 1 2 3 4 DK
  8   The therapist is responsive to the child's direction.0 1 2 3 4 DK
  9   The therapist is responsive to the child's needs.0 1 2 3 4 DK
 10   The therapist is cautious about their interpretations and interventions.0 1 2 3 4 DK
 11   The therapist uses clinically relevant material from the child's life narrative to understand and direct the symbolism in the play.0 1 2 3 4 DK
 12   Total score _____

The FELT format – play analysis through story stems

Perhaps most essential to the FELT format is its use of story stems to structure Play Therapy. There is a rich body of literature on story stems as a means to engage children in structured play. Children's responses to various story stems are then analyzed for content to assess patterns that may differentiate some classes of children from others. For example, the responses of anxious or depressed children can be compared to those of age- and gender-matched "norms" to determine how anxious or depressed children tend to respond to specific stems. This line of research, then, can lead to semi-predictable outcomes in the play of children with various psychiatric concerns.

One of the most well-developed research tools using story stems is the MacArthur Story Stem Battery (MSSB; Emde, Wolfe, & Oppenheim, 2003). The MSSB consists of 14 standard story stems introduced to children using toys. The children are then asked to complete the story as they see fit. Introductions and prompts are highly structured and well-defined in the research protocol, to minimize the likelihood that MSSB-administrators inadvertently change or direct a child's play. After play, stem completions are coded using a structured system.

For example, one of the generalized story stems used in FELT occurs in session 3, which I call the "Robber stem." This stem is used in session 3 to elicit discussion about principles of fear and physiological arousal which can occur in response to certain stimuli. In the Robber stem, the therapist creates a scene in which a child toy is placed in a home alone playing a computer. The therapist shows a father figure leaving to go to work, and then a mother figure is shown telling the child she will be outside working in her garden while the child plays inside on the computer. The therapist has also set up a different room in the home (I often use an "upstairs" portion of a dollhouse, but this can be any room), in which are placed a few valuables. With the scene set, the therapist then introduces two robbers, who break into the room with the valuables. As they are searching for things to steal, they make a noise (e.g., perhaps by knocking something over), which the child hears. The therapist then ends the story stem here and invites the child to continue the story by saying, "What happens next?"[1]

It is in what the child does "next" in finishing story stems that play analysis occurs. In FELT analysis, therapists use a coding system designed after the Narrative Emotion Coding System (NEC), which is an empirically validated system derived from MSSB research (see Warren, 2003). The FELT system is outlined in Table 2.1.

Each of these themes is described in fuller detail, with examples, below.

A preface about coding

In reality, it should be noted that practicing therapists rarely document specific "codes" in any formal manner. In pilot studies, it was found that therapists taking the time to write down codes live in session detracted too much from therapeutic engagement and interfered with continuity of play. In research, sessions were filmed, which allowed for formal coding to occur after sessions and for better analysis of data. However, from a practical standpoint, FELT therapists outside of research settings do not need to generate live

Table 2.1 The FELT play themes

Theme	Description
Initial response	The child's immediate response to the story stem. Coded only as positive or non-positive (negative or neutral).
Final content	How the story ends. Coded as positive, negative, or non-resolution.
Deus ex machina resolution	Occurs when child resolves conflict or affect by simply having it go away, without any indication of what internal or external processes were involved in resolving the problem.
Emotional shift	Any change in emotion that occurs during the play.
Incongruent affect	Displayed or reported affect is inappropriate or incongruent with the story being told.
Reactions to inescapable fear/anxiety	Noted when a child must respond to a stimulus that cannot be or has not yet been escaped. Coded as positive or negative.
Danger	The child maintains, worsens, or introduces danger into the story.
Neediness	The child exhibits a preoccupation with fulfilling (usually basic) needs, such as hunger, sleep, shelter, urinary/bowel needs, etc.
Labeling of emotions and symptoms	The child identifies an emotion by name or identifies symptoms. Coded as present or not present.
Self-representations	Toys or objects the child uses to represent the Self.
"Other" representations	Toys or objects the child uses to represent Others in the child's real life (e.g., family members, the therapist, etc.).

codes of FELT themes or film their sessions for later recording. My and my students' research has also found the 11-code scheme used in FELT is simple enough to be tracked informally and mentally during sessions. In other words, when a child demonstrates neediness or danger, therapists intuitively make note of this and then respond in therapeutic ways. In clinical practice, what matters in FELT is the therapist's *response* to each of these themes, rather than the actual patterns of themes. Patterns matter more in research studies focused on play content.

Additionally, it must be considered that in FELT, therapists are specifically tasked with *intervening* in response to certain themes. From a research perspective, this intervention changes the MSSB-like protocol after which FELT was designed. In the MSSB, researchers specifically do not intervene, which prevents inadvertent interference with data. In FELT, though, therapists *should* intervene, which then presumably changes outcomes. Changing play outcomes, in fact, is the very goal of FELT interventions. Using MSSB data, therapists know what kinds of play outcomes actually differentiate psychiatrically impaired kids from healthy norms (those without any psychiatric complaints). These themes are in a later section of this chapter. Therapists keep these themes in mind and work to drive play to mimic, as closely as possible, that of healthy norms. *It is my belief that the very act of changing play to resemble that of healthy children is a direct therapeutic mechanism of change and is what places FELT decidedly in the Play Therapy (proper) category, because the content of the actual play itself is a direct target of psychotherapy.* Notably, subsequent changes to cognitions and behaviors also do occur and are also targeted, so FELT is also at least partially a cognitive-behavioral therapy. Therapists also target an array of other mechanisms of change, as outlined in Chapter 4, but directly targeting play tends to make up the bulk of the in-session work toward which therapists focus their energies in FELT.

We will now proceed with detailed coverage of the play themes used in FELT play analysis.

Initial response

As indicated in Table 2.1, the child's immediate response to the story stem is coded as the initial response. Usually, therapists limit the noting of this response to its being either positive or non-positive. In the MSSB, codes include positive, negative, and neutral. MSSB research, however, has suggested that negative and neutral responses are functionally equivalent, in that they predict the same outcomes (Emde et al., 2003); thus, in FELT, negative and neutral responses are simplified into a single code – labeled "non-positive." Although therapists make a mental note of a child's initial response, they rarely need to intervene during the immediate response. Although children with anxiety, depression, and other internalizing disorders do tend toward a higher rate of non-positive initial responses compared to healthy norms (Warren, 2003), healthy children do still enjoy at least a small amount of "action" in their play, and thus they tend to tell stories where crises are not necessarily immediately resolved. Furthermore, FELT story stems often purposely leave children at a point of "tension" before they ask the question, "What happens next?" Consequently, this tension leads children to acknowledge the potential for a non-positive initial response, and this isn't always a bad thing. So, I instruct therapists not to become overly concerned about a negative or neutral initial response. Better, therapists should wait and see what happens with the rest of the story.

Final content

Like the initial response, a non-positive final response is an accurate predictor that reliably differentiates anxious from non-anxious children (Warren, 2003). However, whereas therapists may ignore negative or neutral initial responses, they absolutely should make an effort to intervene when a child has completed their story with a non-positive final response. Non-positive final responses can include negative resolutions and non-resolutions. Negative resolutions include a broad array of final outcomes, but basically encompass any non-happy ending to the story. Such endings are hard to define concretely, because they can be so variable, but it is very rare that a therapist is left in doubt, intuitively, about whether an ending is "good" or "bad." Non-resolutions occur when the story or a part of the story has no real end. Sometimes these occur due to time or poor planning by the child. Sometimes kids get distracted and forget to resolve some important part of the story, instead taking the story in a totally different direction. When these errors of omission occur, the therapist can simply help the child re-attend to the core, unresolved portion of the story and work toward some resolution. Other times, children fail to resolve stories because they simply do not know how to resolve them. This often occurs in children who lack coping skills or who lack the imaginal capacity to see how something might end. Therapists can help children develop this capacity, then, by working to direct play toward some kind of at least partially positive resolution.

Regardless of whether the child's ending is negative or a non-resolution, the therapist's task is to engage with the child in various ways to return to the story and work toward a positive ending. Often, this can be done in the same session, where the therapist may invite the child to play again but this time imagine a "happy ending." Or, they may intervene more directly by introducing specific characters or contents into the play that help address weaknesses. For example, in the Robber stem described previously, the child may finish the story by having the child hide in the bathroom, shaking in terror, and afraid to move until the robbers leave. This simple story would constitute a non-resolution, because we do not know how the child feels at all now that the robbers have left, if the child ever emerged from the bathroom, or what they are going to do once their parents come inside and see that a break-in has occurred. Even though the robbers left, there is much in the story still unfinished, so, the therapist may return to the story and start asking the child what they will do now that the robbers are gone. The therapist can then follow the child's lead and, if necessary, suggest getting help from mother and/or calling the police (or a superhero), and work to help continue the story to see if some semblance of safety can be returned to the home. The content of the resolution need not always be realistic. In fact, many children introduce very unrealistic events into the Robber stem. I have seen some children simply go upstairs and overpower the robbers on their own – a reckless, horrible idea to do in the real world, but, through a play, a reflection of self-confidence and personal empowerment that can be quite healthy. Other children have allowed themselves to be kidnapped, only to be later returned home by one of the robbers after they had a change of heart and became "good." In both of these cases, the final content is positive, and thus signifies a movement toward health. So, a therapist's ultimate goal is to facilitate a positive final content when possible, regardless of whether the means to get there are actually feasible in the real world. Practical resolutions are addressed elsewhere (see other codes below).

It is important to note that a therapist will not always be successful at moving a child toward a positive resolution. Some children resist positive resolutions, which can occur for multiple reasons. Occasionally, children simply want to create a somewhat tragic story. This seems to occur more often as children get older and become more aware of other stories (both fictional and real) that end in tragedy. As children read and/or watch more stories, they will eventually become aware that some good stories have tragic endings. Whether it's *Romeo and Juliet* or *Avengers: Endgame*, some storytellers leave audiences without a happy ending, and children are no exception. Thus, a non-positive resolution in spontaneous childhood play is not always a sign for concern, especially for stories whose purpose is to entertain.

Stories in FELT, though, are different. They are not spontaneous and most children understand (at least eventually) that the purpose of the stories is not to entertain. Early in FELT, therapists lay an essential foundation – through play and instruction – that play in FELT is designed to be therapeutic. Furthermore, through interventions as described above, children learn that therapists seem to want stories to have a happy ending. Though some children may be less conscious than others about why we want a happy ending, all children do, eventually, demonstrate a "pull" to execute play according to the therapist's apparent wishes and thus will move play, over time, more reliably toward positive resolutions. Eventually, they build skill in doing this on their own, with less intermediation by the therapist, such that their own, spontaneous play contains more frequent positive resolutions. When this occurs, it can be said that these children are now playing more like healthy, normal children.

So, a child who persistently fails to resolve their play, or who resolves play consistently in a negative manner, is demonstrating two potential important psychological vulnerabilities that must be addressed. In one possibility, children lack the skill to imagine positive resolutions to events. These children tend toward catastrophic thinking in their real lives too. They are pessimistic and seem to feel that if something can go wrong, it will. In children like this, then, the target of play intervention is to help children be able to entertain the possibility of positive resolutions and consider them at least as likely as, if not more likely than, the negative resolution. Through directed play, therapists show these children that positive outcomes can occur, and, in fact, that there are things children can do to focus their attention on the positive outcomes, rather than the negative outcomes.

Another reason children may consistently trend toward negative resolutions is when they become so overwhelmed by "stress" in the play that their coping skills shut down, and they can no longer imagine a way out. This is more likely to happen to children in response to targeted story stems, as these stems are specifically designed to highlight features that concern children in their everyday lives. Resistance in these cases can signify to the therapist that the offending story stem was perhaps too much for the child to handle that day, and thus, the therapist may need to back up, rebuild confidence in coping skills, and then retry the stem again. Sometimes retries can occur in the same session. More often, though, retries occur in later weeks, allowing the child more time to build self-efficacy and confidence. In such cases, therapists simply exercise patience and follow the child's lead with regard to readiness to resolve the difficult scene. Still, resistance to therapist attempts to facilitate a positive resolution to story stems is seen as diagnostic. Resistance should stimulate a diagnostic investigation by the therapist to determine why the child is struggling to rectify a specific scene and what specific coping skills are necessary to generate a healthy resolution.

Deus ex machina *resolution*

In literature, *deus ex machina* literally translates to "God in the machine." The term references a tactic used in ancient Greek tragedies (plays), in which the author, in an attempt to provide relief to the audience at the end of a tragic play, would literally incorporate a device which would lower onto the stage an actor wearing a mask to resemble one of the many Greek gods. This character would then perform some miraculous feat to resolve the tragedy of the play. In modern terms, *deus ex machina*, then, is used as a literary criticism to describe an author who has resorted to "bad writing" to create a resolution of events seemingly out of thin air. There is little attention to whether the resolution fits with the rest of the story or is believable.

In childhood play, *deus ex machina* resolutions are quite common. Children love the fantastic and ridiculous, and so, of course, they will readily employ *deus ex machina* resolutions in their play. Such resolutions are almost always coded as positive final content, and, by definition, do not include non-resolutions. Certainly, there will be times when children will use *deus ex machina* tactics at the end of a story, but the story itself, or important portions of the story, remain unresolved. In these cases, such outcomes are usually coded as non-resolutions and therapists then respond accordingly. A *deus ex machina* resolution, then, is a special case of positive resolution in which a child has demonstrated a lack of knowledge about practical or generalizable coping skills that can be used in the real world. By virtue of being positive, *deus ex machina* resolutions are judged to be better (healthier) than negative or non-resolutions. However, in addition to guiding play toward positive resolutions, therapists also have a responsibility to dedicate time and therapeutic resources to helping children develop translatable, longer-lasting coping skills they may be able to use throughout their lives and across multiple scenarios. So, when a therapist identifies a *deus ex machina* resolution in play, this should usually prompt the therapist to talk with the child about the mechanisms through which the resolution achieved its "calming" purpose in the play.

Let's take the following example, once again using the Robber stem. Let's imagine that a child continued the Robber stem by having the robbers kidnap the child and hold them for ransom. The parents are unable to pay the ransom and seek help from the police. Police attempt to recover the child, but they are killed in the process. The parents call another police officer, and this officer is also killed by the robbers/kidnappers. Next, the parents decide to take matters into their own hands and attempt a rescue of their own. They also are killed. Meanwhile, the child becomes increasingly frightened, locked inside a cage. One day, the robbers leave the child alone in the cage as they go "rob some more stuff." While alone, the child prays for help. Immediately after prayer, the door magically opens, and the child is able to escape. They go to visit their parents' dead bodies, which are still just outside the building where the child was being held. The child casts a magic spell and their parents are resurrected from the dead. Together, the child and the parents decide to build a trap which will lock the robbers/kidnappers/murderers in the same cage in which the child was locked. The bad guys return, and the trap works. They are caught in their own cage. The family calls the police again, and the police come and take the robbers and put them in a triple cage they can never break out of. The story ends there.

In this story, quite a lot has happened, and there are quite a few codes we could list, including some we have not explored yet. Of those we have defined, *initial content* is negative (the child is kidnapped). *Final content* is positive. The content of the story has been largely resolved. An astute, experienced FELT therapist may note that although content has been resolved, there was no mention of how emotions were resolved. The child was frightened at some point in the story, but we don't know if they are still frightened now that the bad guys are locked away. We don't know if they may get frightened again once they return home and/or see other traumatic triggers for the experience. These are features the therapist would want to address eventually. However, a therapist may also note a (fairly literal, in this case) *deus ex machina* resolution when the child prayed to God and was miraculously saved from their captivity and then was able to revive the dead parents. In this example, though, the therapist should not feel a need to take a stance toward a more "realistic" outcome of the play. The issue here is not the "realism" of the play but the lack of detail about the mechanisms of recovery from the stressful events. So, to help explore mechanisms, the therapist may ask how the child's prayer helped. They may then look for themes in the response such as intercession from a higher power/authority (e.g., "I asked for help and God helped me"), social support/comfort (e.g., "I felt God was with me, and I felt safe"), or cognitive restructuring (e.g., "I told myself everything would be alright"). All of these are positive coping skills characterizing healthy children and can translate to generalizable real-world skills. Thus, therapists can highlight these themes in the mechanisms of a *deus ex machina* resolution.

In summary, then, a *deus ex machina* resolution is a positive resolution, generally seen as a good sign more consistent with healthy than unhealthy children. However, such resolutions should prompt therapists to help the child identify specific mechanisms and coping skills enhanced by the *deus ex machina* technique. When they see a *deus ex machina* resolution, therapists need not worry about feasibility of the actual resolution in real-world practice, but rather should focus on highlighting what specific coping skills occurred as a result of the resolution.

Emotional shift

Emotional shifts are quite frequent in childhood play, albeit they are not always explicit. In fact, most spontaneous childhood play mentions rather little about emotions at all. Consequently, emotional shifts are often inferred and then subsequently discovered by the therapist after prompting a child to label emotions across the shift. Naturally, children tend to focus much more heavily on external content/behaviors of characters, rather than their internal states (unless prompted to do so). So, emotional shifts are most often first suspected and then confirmed through collaboration with the child.

It is for this reason that emotional shifts are noted by therapists, not because of their inherent importance, per se, to play analysis, but rather because they can signify a need to prompt a child to better label what emotions are actually occurring. If we take the example given in the previous section on *deus ex machina* resolutions, it is notable that several emotional shifts probably occurred in between being kidnapped and held captive (i.e., presumably fear/anxiety increased over this time), when police and parents were killed (more fear; perhaps despair; hopelessness), and then when the door opened and the child was again safe, and the kidnappers were captured (perhaps some relief). In this example, the therapist can use content of the play to infer that some kind of emotional shift likely occurred, but the therapist must then confirm these suspicions by investigating with the child. Thus, as they are intervening as described above to explore mechanisms of change and coping skills, therapists can use emotional shifts as focal points to note what emotions trigger a need for different coping skills. These connections help children build self-awareness for using those coping skills in similar, more generalized situations outside of play. By calling attention to the emotional shift, therapists are showing children that it is this shift that triggers the need for a coping skill, not the actual event itself. Children are unlikely to actually be kidnapped and experience the horrific events of the play scene described, but they are very likely to routinely feel fear, anxiety, despair, hopelessness, and any other emotions elicited by the play scene. By helping children focus on the emotions and emotional shifts, therapists help generalize what happens in these play scenes to more typical real-world scenarios.

Still, not all emotional shifts warrant an immediate response from therapists. Instead, often it helps for therapists to watch numerous shifts over several play scenes and sessions before deciding how and when to intervene. Doing so allows a more generalized sample of a child's general emotional content, which then translates to better hypotheses about how to target emotional shifts, and which ones need targeting the most. For example, I once worked with a six-year-old child (and she is just one example, there are many others like her) who, in one of her first play scenes, was instructed to show me a "happy time." She decided to re-enact a recent trip to Disney World, and her scene shifted from apprehension ("What will it be like?"), to joy, to uncontrollable excitement, to sleepiness, to fear (she was afraid of fireworks), to disappointment (when it was time to leave), and finally to gratitude, thanking her parents for taking her. That is six emotional shifts in just one scene, which is a lot of ground to cover for anyone, much less for a six-year-old. In deciding how to respond to these, I focused back on the goals for the session (in this case, the first session), which are focused on building rapport and demonstrating how play will be used throughout therapy. Because we were early in treatment, I did not yet know well the girl's specific pre-existing coping skills or her general play style. So, highlighting every emotional shift that occurred in this scene was beyond the scope of the current session. Instead, I decided just to note the shifts in general ("Sometimes big, exciting things give us a lot of different feelings, don't they?") and then I chose a few to highlight to get her to tell or show me again what those feelings were like. Since this is a "happy time" scene, I chose a happy, positive emotion ("When you were happy, how did you show it in your body? In your face? With your words?"). I also highlighted how a single emotion can come at different levels ("At the beginning, you were pretty excited, and then you got REALLY excited, and then it went back down to just a happy"). As I will note later in this book when I review the actual goals of each session, these reactions/statements are guided by specific session goals. Emotional shifts, because they are so common, are among the more frequent themes to which a therapist may respond differently depending on specific session goals. Overall, the take-home message of this section is that emotional shifts serve as markers for points of intervention according to session goals.

Incongruent affect

Sometimes, in play and in life, children display emotions that do not match the surrounding environment or context. Incongruent affect exists as a code to capture when these moments occur in FELT. Like emotional shifts, incongruent affect serves as a marker to identify points of further analysis. FELT stems are specifically designed to elicit certain types of possible emotional responses. The Robber stem is designed to elicit fear – a healthy child should be quite afraid if their house is invaded while they are home alone. If a child showed no sign of fear in this situation, incongruent affect would be coded. A curious therapist, then, should want to know why the child eschewed fear in this scene. Importantly, not every scene of incongruent affect is an active avoidance tactic. It is tempting for therapists to assume that if a child denies fear in an obvious fear-inducing situation, they must be engaging in avoidance, which must mean they are "afraid" to admit weakness or that they are not in touch with their true emotions. Certainly, avoidance is a valid *possible* interpretation of incongruent affect, but other possibilities must be considered as well. Sometimes, incongruent affect is just a display of confidence and security. A child who is unafraid of the robbers in play may be simply demonstrating the normal narcissism associated with early childhood (see Chapter 3). Believing themselves to be invincible, such a child may confront the robbers alone and subdue them with ease. If the therapist interprets such play as being a demonstration of normal narcissism, they may then respond as healthy parents do to similar exhibitionist displays of childhood – with awe, wonder, and by building up the child's sense of Self. "Wow! You really handled those bad guys! You are so brave and so strong!"

Next, the therapist may then refocus the child toward the goal of the stem – that is, the elicitation and exploration of fear. The therapist may return to the scene and suggest playing again, imagining what would happen if the child were too afraid to fight the robbers alone. In this intervention, the therapist has allowed room to follow the child's own initial response to the stem, but they are also using their expertise to return attention to the child's therapeutic needs.

So, incongruent affect typically needs two things: 1) therapists' attention to session goals and desired outcomes for a session, and 2) an analytic mind to identify potential reasons for the incongruent affect. In my experience developing FELT and teaching it to numerous other therapists over the years, I have found the following common reasons that children show incongruent affect.

1   Childhood innocence: by far the most common reason for incongruent affect is that children routinely display incongruent affect in their everyday lives. They rarely understand the seriousness and implications of real-world events, and, as such, tend to overlook negative components of the world around them. This tendency is further enhanced in fantasy play, because children understand that the play is not real, and, thus, they become even more likely to remove the seriousness from play scenes. So, if a stressful event is happening in play, and the child shows no signs of distress, more often than not this is done simply out of a child's confidence and desire to allow the story to resolve happily. As we will note in Chapter 3, children (especially young children) are naturally driven toward optimism, and this optimism can sometimes present as incongruent affect in play. When innocence/optimism is the reason for

incongruent affect, the therapist's role in most cases is to respond by attempting to introduce "realistic" emotional responses in other play characters. Depending on the child's stage/progress in therapy too, the therapist can adapt the intensity and persistence of these "realistic" reactions. In the beginning of therapy, these emotions may be relatively light and easily resolved. The therapist may even have to model how to resolve them through the play, but therapists in initial sessions should generally allow their characters' introduced emotions to be resolved easily, which can help promote momentum and hope in the child that resolution is possible. As a child progresses through therapy, however, and as they have learned a wider array of coping skills, therapists can execute a role reversal, where the therapist enacts the stressed/anxious character and the child takes the role of coaching that character through therapeutic healing. Such role reversals help children develop mastery over generalizable coping skills. In late therapy, therapists may even resist some of the "simpler" fixes introduced by children, pressing them to use more realistic or varied coping skills to manage a stressful situation. In following the above steps, therapists are not "correcting" the child's normal innocence, but rather are demonstrating that other responses are also possible and manageable.

2   Anxious avoidance: research tells us that people with clinically significant anxiety/distress tend to engage in anxious avoidance. More specifically, they not only avoid anxiety-provoking situations; they also avoid the stressful/anxious feelings. The very emotion of stress/anxiety is seen as a dire state which must be evaded. So, many children may skim over negative affect in play because they are (consciously or unconsciously) avoiding the negative emotion. In these cases, a therapist responds similarly to other descriptions above, by refocusing the child in some way toward the negative emotion through play. There is no need in Play Therapy to directly confront a child's incongruent affect. It is ill-advised to challenge a child, saying, "You don't have to pretend not to be scared," or, "Don't avoid your feelings." Rather, therapists *show* children these feelings through play, and they also show how the feelings can be managed/resolved safely.

3   Hyper/Unfocused annulment: although some are more prone to doing so than others, all children can become distracted during play. It has happened to us all as therapists. We've worked to prepare the most incredible story stem, perfectly suited to our clients' needs. We're so proud of it and can't wait to use it with our client. Then, we go into session, start our story stem, and we find we've got a child who for some reason today is psychologically (or physically) all over the place. They are not so hyper/unfocused that no work can get done (if that were the case, the therapist might need to transition to a more behaviorally focused treatment designed for children with disruptive behavior disorders (e.g., ADHD)).

They can be still enough to engage in play, but their play skips from one scene to another and they take your story in some completely unforeseen direction, moving so quickly that they are hard to follow. By the end of the story, you feel you've lost control of the play and have no idea how you and your child even arrived at the end you got to. This play is considered a hyper/unfocused annulment because the child's lack of focus has essentially dissolved your plans for that scene. It is a version of incongruent affect because in their dissolution of the scene, they also tend to display inconsistent and/or unpredictable emotional content.

4   When (not if) this happens to you, it is important not to lose your bearings or beat yourself up. The best course of action is to attempt to ground the child and try again. If it's temporary (only one session and atypical of the child), attribute it to an erratic day for the child (everyone has them) and perhaps try again next session. If it happens routinely, you'll need to treat the lack of focus before you can be effective with Play Therapy, and therapists are advised to use other evidence-based methods improving childhood focus/attention.

5   Sometimes, it may be the story itself causing the unfocused annulment. When unfocused annulment occurs, therapists are advised to question whether their story stem may have caused it. Perhaps the setting or content of the story was too "exciting" for this particular child, and so a change in the story content may help address the annulment. Other story stems may be too complex for children and will need to be simplified or abbreviated to allow less room for deviation from the goal. In such cases, a modest change in story stem can do the trick for bringing children back into a productive session.

Reactions to inescapable fear/anxiety

Many children escape stressful scenes in play by simply making the stressor "go away." Though eliminating stressors is fine in play, it does not always translate well to the real world. So, therapists will typically need, at some point in therapy, to introduce story stems that present an inescapable type of stressor. The goal of these stems is to force children to actively manage anxiety/fear/worry, learning to appreciate that such emotions are healthy and need not be always avoided, but, rather, modulated. One inescapable story stem I use often is a Storm stem. In the Storm stem, I usually set up children at their home or school and then announce that a tornado or other severe, damaging storm is passing through the neighborhood. I then work with the children to identify, explore, and then modulate any anxieties that arise as a result of the storm.

Responses to these inescapable stimuli are coded in two core categories: 1) successful emotion modulation, and 2) failed emotion modulation. Failed emotion modulation typically presents in three types: a) escape, b) avoidance, or c) defeat. In escape, children persist in trying to eliminate or escape the stressor. In a tornado stem, for example, they make the tornado just disappear without causing any damage or they call in Superman who blows the storm away with his super-breath. In avoidance, children allow the stressor to stay, but deny any fear or anxiety about the stressor. Even as the tornado passes right overhead, these children insist none of the children in the story have any fear. In defeat, children allow the stressor and acknowledge the fear, but they do not cope with it and never resolve the fear. In my experience, defeat is the worst kind of failure because it represents a complete lack of confidence in positive outcomes. In other words, whereas escape and avoidance usually still lead to a positive resolution, defeat is nearly always a negative or non-positive resolution.

The therapist's response to each of the above is similar to that described in other themes. If the child attempts escape, the therapist can simply disallow the escape and challenge the child to label and describe what feelings are present in various characters, then work to resolve them as needed. The therapist can assume roles as needed by inserting worry/fear into other characters, if the child does not do so themselves. Similarly, if avoidance is noted, the therapist responds as described previously in other types of avoidance. In defeat, therapists respond as they would for any other non-positive resolution. Altogether, then, this code exists not so much to differentiate a therapist's response to other story stem content, but, rather, to highlight that therapists must choose, at some point, to challenge a child by pushing them to face a fear they cannot just escape and then note how their response in that scenario may differ from less challenging story stems.

Danger

Many children love to introduce danger into their story stems. Most often, danger is a manifestation of a child's attempt to make the story more interesting. It is a storytelling tactic, and nothing more. For this reason, therapists need not necessarily respond immediately to all danger codes in a child client's play. Still, research has shown that children with externalizing behavior problems (e.g., symptoms of ADHD, Oppositional Defiant Disorder (ODD), and/or Conduct Disorder) as rated by parents exhibit higher frequencies of danger than healthy norms (Warren, 2003). These findings lead some play therapists to want to decrease danger in play as a means to normalize play, which presumably would then translate to increased health. However, I find that a strict play-based approach is ill-suited for efficient management of primary childhood externalizing symptoms. Rather, behavior therapy and parent management training are much stronger options for treating externalizing symptoms (see Weisz & Kazdin, 2017). My argument, then, is successful treatment of externalizing symptoms decreases danger in play, but decreasing danger in play does not successfully treat externalizing symptoms. So, in most cases, I advise therapists to ignore isolated instances of danger to allow the story to "play out."

Nevertheless, danger can be meaningful when it attaches to other codes/ themes as a hint to what triggers various responses. For example, some therapists may note that a child routinely omits labeling of emotions during or immediately after a danger code. Similarly, some children may pair danger with neediness (see below), which can clue therapists toward emotional triggers and other emotional shifts. So, in FELT, danger is coded mainly as a marker to guide analysis of other themes and to aid in the individualized case conceptualization.

Neediness

Neediness is coded when a child displays a preoccupation with fulfilling (basic) needs such as eating, sleeping, toileting, shelter, etc. It is not uncommon for children to play out domestic scenes that may involve all basic needs. Like danger, many times, the introduction of domestic rituals in play is a storytelling tactic. It is also just a manifestation of children enacting through play events that occur in their daily life. Domestic play is also prompted by toy selection. If your play materials include a dollhouse with furniture, including kitchen, bedroom, and bathroom, children are likely to play with these in the intended way. Thus, just because a child plays a domestic scene does not mean neediness has occurred. Rather, neediness is coded only when meeting these needs becomes a core focus of a particular story. Neediness also need not be overt. While some children may exhibit clear and obvious neediness – looking everywhere for food, trying to sleep but being unable to, wetting themselves and needing a diaper change – others may do so more subtly, perhaps by repeatedly and perseveratively eating or going to bed or going "potty," without ever experiencing satisfaction. So, neediness encapsulates two broad categories of content: 1) dependence (on others), and 2) unsatisfaction (of needs).

Dependent neediness is healthy in many cases. MSSB research, for example, found that one feature that differentiates the play of anxious versus healthy kids is that healthy kids more readily seek help from a parent or adult figure in play, whereas anxious children attempt more often to solve problems on their own (Warren, 2003). Some may see this finding as counterintuitive. Especially in US culture, independent children are usually judged to be more mature than their counterparts, and thus higher functioning overall. So, many would assume that themes of independence in play would also translate to higher functioning. In reality though, children who are overly independent often persist in trying to solve problems alone even when they do not have the skills to do so. They resist aid from adult or other more mature helpers. Healthy children, on the other hand, seek help, or, at the very least, they welcome help when it is offered. So, at proper levels, dependence is healthy.

Where dependence becomes unhealthy is if the child seems to passively await help without doing enough to increase the likelihood that help will come. This form of neediness is characterized by children who cower in the bathroom during the Robber stem, petrified by fear, or who cry out in hunger for mother to come feed them, but who do not go to get mother if she does not hear or does not come. Sure, crying is an action in this example, but the key is whether or not the action actually succeeded in meeting the need. If it did not (as in this case, since mother did not hear when the child cried), neediness can be coded.

Unsatisfied neediness overlaps quite a bit with dependent neediness. In fact, in the example above (child crying for mother, but mother does not come), there is both dependence ("I need mother") and unsatisfaction ("but she did not come"). This is one of the reasons there are not formal "subcodes" for neediness, because there is so much overlap that differentiating them is not always possible. Still, unsatisfied neediness is designed to capture both single actions that are unsuccessful in meeting a goal as well as all types of play where a child repeats an identical action more than once. The presumption in the latter case is that by virtue of repeating the action, the child is suggesting that the first time was unsatisfying/unsuccessful and is thus expressing some sort of unsatisfied need. In research settings, neediness would be coded with every subsequent repetition of the same action. So, if a child sends their character to the toilet seven times during a session, six codes of neediness are coded for each instance after the first (technically, the "counts" are for the first six instances, with the final repetition assumed to be the one that finally satisfied the need). In clinical settings, such detailed quantitative measures are rarely feasible, but therapists should notice multiple repetitions and may interpret increased repetitions as being indicative of increased unsatisfied neediness.

When unsatisfied repetitions occur, therapists are triggered to try to identify the unmet need. Therapists can use Maslow's hierarchy of needs (Maslow, 1943) as a general guide for the types of needs to monitor. Once the therapist hypothesizes the specific need, they then test the hypothesis through commentary. If we take the crying child example given before, the therapist may comment reflectively, "This baby wants his mommy to feed him, but she didn't come. What a sad baby! Will mommy ever come?" In this case, the therapist hypothesizes logically that the child wants mother not just for food/hunger but also for love and comfort. For this reason, the therapist highlighted how "sad" the baby was, rather than focusing only on hunger. Through this subtle comment, the therapist is suggesting to the child that humans rely on others not just for basic physical needs but also for emotional needs. They are also leaving room for the child to explore emotions and how they can be resolved in this instance. So, by noticing the child's neediness, hypothesizing about the cause(s) of the neediness, and then purposefully structuring commentary to highlight key therapeutic points, the therapist pushes attention toward key therapeutic issues that need resolution. Then, of course, when possible, they work to help the child achieve resolution of the need.

Labeling of emotions and symptoms

Labeling is among the simpler codes in FELT, as it is fairly self-explanatory. Therapists simply code whether some sort of direct or indirect emotional labeling has occurred or not. Labeling includes not only naming specific emotions present, but also describing the emotions through physiological or psychological symptoms. So, a child may label a character as being "sad," or they may state the character "feels heavy and wants to cry because no one wants to play with them." In the latter case, there is an implication that the character is sad and/or lonely, which can be confirmed and refined through simple reflection, "Oh man! I hate feeling lonely too!"

Therapists always want labeling to occur, and so when it is absent, therapists are guided to return to play to promote labeling, but therapists should usually not interrupt a flowing narrative in order to force labeling to occur at every moment, especially if the child struggles with simple prompts. Instead, it is better to follow the child's narrative through to the end and then return to label emotions and symptoms later. In the example above, the therapist commented, "Oh man! I hate feeling lonely too!" In my experience, most children do not respond verbally to these types of reflective comments. They may make eye contact and smile at you, but they usually will not offer clear verbal affirmation that your interpretation is correct (they will, however, more often correct you if you are wrong, "No, he's not lonely. He's mad!"). If the child doesn't really "bite" at the brief comment, let them finish the story and make a mental note to come back later and invite the child to explore that loneliness a bit more deeply. A similar action is warranted with direct labeling. If the child says the character is "sad," a therapist may ask in the moment, "What does sad feel like?" but if the child does not provide a satisfactory response right away, it is not necessary to persist in the moment in getting a more detailed description of sadness. Rather, detailed labeling can occur after the conclusion of the story.

Self-representations

Simple in concept, but somewhat complicated in practice, Self-representations are the characters in play that represent the child's Self. Many times, a child's Self-toys are obvious. In fact, in the first session, the therapist explicitly instructs the child to select some toys that tell the therapist about the child, in which case all selections are obvious Self-toys. Other times, though, Self-toys are less obvious, and some therapists can even make erroneous assumptions about the Self-toy. Children rarely explicitly tell therapists, "This toy is just like me" (though it does happen). For this reason, therapists are almost always making interpretive *guesses* about their clients' Self-toys, based on what makes the most sense with the child's case conceptualization, combined with some leading by the therapist. FELT story stems are designed for the child to identify with specific characters in the play, and so FELT therapists often lead children toward specific Self-toys in play, which aids in interpretation. This is another way in which the structure of FELT story stems aids in interpretation. In free play, identifying which characters represent whom is more difficult. Still, the Self-toy is not always clear, and so it is imperative for therapists to exercise caution and make only tentative guesses when analyzing Self-toy content.

Self-representations are a more variable (open-ended) qualitative code, compared to the other FELT themes. In research/statistical terms, other FELT codes are qualified as closed, nominal data, codable in spreadsheets with 0s (absent) and 1s (present) and readily usable for advanced logistic analyses. Self-representations (and their companion, "Other" representations) are unique, though, in that they are not codified as if to be used in logistic statistical models. Instead, they are designed more similarly to axial coding techniques used in grounded theory as it applies to qualitative research (see Birks & Mills, 2015). For those unfamiliar with qualitative research methodologies, this simply means that a ready-made coding system for Self-representations is not used in FELT. Rather, therapists closely analyze Self-representations in context and over time (preferably a minimum of 15–30 different Self-representations) to gather ideas about the child's sense of Self and how that links with psychopathology and with other themes presented during FELT.

Still, clinical experience with FELT and additional research can highlight some core ideas to look for in child Self-representations. Particularly salient is general self-competence. MSSB research (Warren, 2003) has shown that children with incompetent or insufficiently competent Self-representations tend also to be rated by others as having anxious symptoms. Thus, a Self-toy with low competence is a sign of psychopathology which should trigger the therapist to remedy. Consequently, therapists should make a point to look in particular at competence in Self-representations.

Similarly, the same research also showed, as indicated previously, that anxious children tend to display overly independent Self-toys (those who take on parental roles or seek to do too much themselves). Thus, because we already know of this empirical association, therapists are instructed to intervene when children display overly independent selves.

Taking these research data into account, and considering clinical and research experience with FELT so far, I recommend therapists seek to answer the following relevant questions about a child's Self-representations:

1 What is their competence to solve the problems presented in story stems? Do perceived competencies match objectively rated competencies and normal developmental expectations?
2 Do they seek help from others when needed? If so, how do they prefer to seek help?
3 What is the general valence of the depicted global Self (positive or negative)?

4   Are there specific strengths and/or weaknesses depicted? If so, what are they? If not, why not (developmental reasons, avoidance, lack of opportunity to show them in story stems so far, etc.)?
5   What is the nature of peer relationships shown in play? What do peer relationships suggest about attitudes toward the Self?
6   How does the Self respond to danger? Is the response different to various types or levels of danger? Does the "target" of the danger matter?
7   How does the Self meet its own needs?
8   How does the Self meet Others' needs?
9   How does the Self respond to Others' attempts to provide for the child's needs?
10 How do any Self-representations fit into the FELT case conceptualization for this child?

Chapter 3, on Object-relations theory in FELT, provides a useful framework for understanding the importance of these questions in categorizing a child's overall Self-development and then working in therapy to move it toward healthy norms.

"Other" representations

"Other" representations involve any other characters that are not Self-representations. Their process for coding and their purpose are identical to Self-representations. As a guide for interpreting "Other" representations, I find it helpful to also understand *archetypes*, and to keep in mind the basic cultural archetypes that are relevant to the lives of children. In FELT, archetypes signify classifications of Objects into general categories depending on their purpose. Many students of psychology associate archetypes with Carl Jung and the 12 Jungian archetypes, which are also associated with the concept of the "collective unconscious." FELT practitioners need not be intimately familiar with Jungian theory to effectively administer FELT. Instead, a few basic requisite ideas are sufficient to utilize archetypes in analysis. First, FELT does hold to be true the idea that human beings as a whole possess an innate need to cognitively classify Others into meaningful "prototypes," and these prototypes do have a greater cultural definition that goes above and beyond individualized ideas of Others. For example, regardless of what kind of mother a person actually has, that person also internalizes the cultural sense that a mother is supposed to embody certain prototypical features, namely, nurturance, kindness, loving, etc. Similarly, each person forms an archetypal understanding of "father" from larger societal definitions, which usually includes "provider, protector, and playmate," among other things. Thus, FELT assumes that children possess and are actively developing archetypes based on their experiences of Others and based on accepted broader societal definitions.

In FELT, the following archetypes are generally seen to be useful in play analysis:

1 Mother
2 Father
3 Hero/Good guy
4 Villain/Bad guy
5 Friend
6 Doctor/Healer
7 Protector/Defender
8 Teacher/Guide/Coach
9 Pet (this is an archetype like "Friend," but there is also a sense of ownership over the Object, with a hierarchy that the "owner" rules over and/ or takes care of the pet).

FELT therapists are instructed to monitor for representations of each of the above archetypes in FELT, primarily for use in the child's individual case conceptualization. Analysis of "Other" representations does not require immediate action or response in most cases, although therapists may at times choose to correct distorted "Other" representations if the representations seem to contribute to or derive from psychopathology. For example, some children may depict all teachers/guides/coaches as bad guys, which would be an extreme classification not consistent with reality. So, the therapist may help to introduce teachers/guides/coaches that display healthier characteristics, as an example to the child that not all teachers/guides/coaches are so bad.

Again, the review of Object-relations theory outlined in Chapter 3 provides more information about the connections between internal representations of Others (Objects) and mental health.

The prime maladaptive themes

Childhood play offers the potential for extremely rich analytic content, and given FELT does include 11 themes, it is possible that therapists can sometimes "get lost in the data" within a single live session. FELT uses a somewhat reduced coding system (the 11 themes) compared to other, research-based structures (some of which use 50+ or even 100+ codes), and so it is designed to be simple and usable in a live therapy session (rather than saving coding for later video review). Nonetheless, even tracking these 11 codes can lead therapists in multiple directions at once, unsure where to intervene or how to immediately respond. So, in this section, I review a summary of core ideas that guide therapeutic decision-making in FELT. A therapist should always keep these core ideas in mind, and, when stuck, should focus therapeutic interventions toward resolving these ideas. Because these three themes are considered to be the most important in FELT, I call them the "prime" themes, here.

The prime maladaptive themes were derived from MSSB-related research summarized previously (see also Emde et al., 2003). These play themes occur more often in children with (anxious) psychopathology compared to those without. Because FELT was designed originally as an anxiety-focused treatment, and because FELT-supportive studies so far have all focused on children with anxiety disorders, the maladaptive themes of focus in FELT are those which identify clinically anxious children. However, it is my belief, which is consistent with other treatments of anxiety, depression, and other types of negative affect, that FELT principles and maladaptive themes can apply to any form of negative affect. In fact, it can be argued that the true target of FELT treatment is not anxiety, per se, but negative affect. So, the official FELT position is that the following maladaptive core themes are representative of negative affect, and should thus be remedied in treatment.[2] The core maladaptive themes include 1) non-positive initial content, 2) non-positive final content, and 3) incompetent Self-representations. If a therapist can keep these in mind throughout FELT, and can then intervene accordingly, they will have a high likelihood of success with the program.

As indicated above, however, we have found through initial FELT research that intervention during a non-positive initial content is inessential and typically causes more interference, than aid, in children's play. In other words, stopping or changing play at the point of initial content is seen to be counterproductive, because doing so either then changes the rest of the play content (which may not always be desirable) or it doesn't (in which case the therapist has done the equivalent of nothing). In both cases, the outcome is rarely as desirable as alternatives, and so it is better to simply note initial content but allow play to continue.

Once noted, however, initial content can be a useful point of intervention when repeating story stems and working toward healthier resolutions. So, let us imagine, for example, a child who completed a story stem with both a negative initial and negative final content. In this case, the therapist will want to help play resolve in a more positive manner, and one way they may do so is by repeating the stem and then intervening immediately at the initial content. Then, the therapist can "back off" a bit and see how the child responds to the now more positive initial content. Most children respond by then improving the rest of the play. They follow the lead/momentum and carry the play toward a final resolution. This can be powerful for children, because they are acting on the boost, but are mostly doing the work themselves to bring about a positive resolution. So, even though therapists rarely react to an initial content in a first-time play-through of a story, they should still note the initial content so that they can intervene accordingly in any repetitions.

The other two core maladaptive themes are negative final content and incompetent Self-representations, each of which is reviewed in detail above. If a therapist accomplishes nothing else in a therapy session, driving the play toward a positive final content and doing so in a way that boosts a child's self-competence are the prime goals of every session. Thus, all interventions implemented by the therapist should be focused toward these prime goals. The remaining themes/goals are secondary. Still, accomplishing the prime goals is not believed to be sufficient to cause real, lasting change in children. Building and honing lifelong coping skills typically requires some attention toward the remaining themes as well.

FELT designed as a treatment for anxiety

Though it has already been stated that FELT was designed as a treatment for anxiety, it is important to note how research goals influenced the design of FELT in its current state and how they have limited the empirical generalizability of FELT so far. Because FELT was specifically created to fill an empirical gap in the Play Therapy literature, I purposefully incorporated several features of research design that improve empirical rigor and facilitate reliability and validity of data.

Using story stems and structured FELT themes were both part of the empirical nature of FELT. I needed a play therapy that used predictable, repeatable play scenes and analysis, while still allowing flexibility in following a child's lead in play. I also needed a population of children with whom to explore if FELT would actually work the way it was intended. As I considered different possible conditions to treat, there were a few that a) were readily available in the setting in which I worked, and b) included the age range of children I needed (ages 4–12). These conditions included anxiety, depression, trauma, and ADHD. I was able to nix ADHD somewhat readily. The evidence-based treatments for ADHD are decidedly behavioral, with individual therapy rarely being offered (except for treating co-morbid emotional conditions), and I did not want to create another behavior therapy. This left me with anxiety, depression, and trauma. I excluded depression because there were no other existing treatments for children ages 4–12 with depression (and there really still aren't) (see Weisz & Kazdin, 2017). One of the main reasons for this is because young children are rarely diagnosed with depression. More often, pediatric depression presents differently than adolescent or adult depression, with significant symptom overlap with anxiety and/or anger/irritability. For this, and other complex reasons, it has been nearly impossible so far in the history of psychotherapy research to establish a clear treatment specifically for early-to-middle-childhood depression, and I felt at the time that diving into such a complex treatment deficit for a time-limited major research project was beyond the scope of what I could or should do for a dissertation project. So, I ruled out depression.[3]

My remaining options were now anxiety and trauma. There is already considerable overlap in the treatment of anxiety and trauma, with the main difference being that trauma incorporates more direct trauma-related exposures and trauma-related narratives. Otherwise, though, the two treatments progress very similarly. Likewise, the empirical support for anxiety-focused and trauma-focused treatments is fairly identical, with each having quite robust support for CBT. However, in the setting in which I was working, the children with trauma-related psychiatric needs nearly all had complex trauma (see Ford & Courtois, 2009), as opposed to acute trauma. Complex trauma is difficult to categorize, symptomatically variable, and typically requires longer-term treatment compared to acute trauma and/or anxiety. My research goals at the time limited me to a confined data collection period, which did not leave me with the one to two years of treatment typically recommended for the types of complex trauma present in my clinical setting at the time. Thus, given my research goals – to develop an empirically supportable form of Play Therapy, comparable to forms of therapy already used (i.e., CBT), and researchable in typical clinical settings – I selected children with anxiety disorders as my population of interest.

Because I selected the anxiety-disordered population, though, for my sample, I then needed to create FELT specifically to fit the needs of the selected population. Thus, FELT was designed purposefully to treat clinically significant anxiety. The themes were included and written to capture anxious functioning, as were the story stems themselves. Case conceptualization is based on etiological models of pediatric anxiety. Outcomes also focused on anxiety and anxious symptoms.

Still, my goal with FELT was never to establish another empirically supported treatment for children with anxiety. Though I have now done the research (see Steadman, 2016) to market FELT as an emerging empirically supported treatment (EST) for anxiety, and though I want therapists to be able to use FELT for anxious children when it fits, I also, more importantly, want FELT, and this book, to serve as a model for designing similar researchable, play-based treatments for other childhood disorders. I believe that story stems and structured thematic analysis are the keys to moving Play Therapy toward a stronger empirical basis, and I believe that other clinicians and researchers can use the lessons throughout this book to develop other programs for children suffering from a greater variety of psychiatric illnesses – depression, trauma, and other stress-related disorders included – with condition-specific adaptations (to the etiological model used in case conceptualization, to the measured outcomes, and to the actual story stem content) being made according to need.

Notes

1 It should be noted that by this point in therapy, the child has already seen several previous story stems and understands the general structure – that they are to wait until the stem is complete and then they can take over and complete the stem however they wish.
2 Empirically speaking, though, FELT has only been evaluated with anxiety. Formal studies so far have excluded children with depression, trauma, or any other primary

cause of negative affect, although I have used some of the techniques with other, general sources of negative affect in my practice.

3   As discussed in Chapter 12, though, adapting FELT for depression remains a goal for future research.

REFERENCES

Axline, V. M. (1974). *Play Therapy*. New York: Ballantine Books.

Birks, M., & Mills, J. (2015). *Grounded Theory: A Practical Guide* (2nd ed.). London: Sage.

Bratton, S. C., Ray, D., Rhine, T., & Jones, L. (2005). The efficacy of play therapy with children: a meta-analytic review of treatment outcomes. *Professional Psychology: Research and Practice*, 36(4), 376–390.

Emde, R. N., Wolfe, D. P., & Oppenheim, D. (2003). *Revealing the Inner Worlds of Young Children: The MacArthur Story Stem Battery and Parent-Child Narratives*. Oxford: Oxford University Press.

Ford, J. D., & Courtois, C. A. (2009). Defining and understanding complex trauma and complex traumatic stress disorders. In C. A. Courtois & J. D. Ford (Eds.), *Treating Complex Traumatic Stress Disorders: An Evidence-Based Guide* (pp. 13–30). New York: Guilford.

Higa-McMillan, C. K., Francis, S. E., Rith-Najarian, L., & Chorpita, B. F. (2016). Evidence base update: 50 years of research on treatment for child and adolescent anxiety. *Journal of Clinical Child and Adolescent Psychology*, 45(2), 91–113.

Johnson, J. L. (2016). The history of play therapy. In K. J. O'Connor, C. E. Schaefer, & L. D. Braverman (Eds.), *Handbook of Play Therapy* (pp. 17–34). Hoboken, NJ: Wiley.

Maslow, A. H. (1943). A theory of human motivation. *Psychological Review*, 50(4), 370–396.

O'Connor, K. J., Schaefer, C. E., & Braverman, L. D. (Eds.). (2016). *Handbook of Play Therapy*. Hoboken, NJ: Wiley.

Phillips, R. D. (2010). How firm is our foundation? Current play therapy research. *International Journal of Play Therapy*, 19(1), 13–25.

Steadman, J. (2016). Evidence-based practice in play-analysis: interpreting and using the play of anxious children. *British Journal of Play Therapy*, 12, 52–75.

Warren, S. L. (2003). Narrative emotion coding system (NEC). In R. N. Emde, D. P. Wolfe, & D. Oppenheim (Eds.), *Revealing the Inner Worlds of Young Children: The MacArthur Story Stem Battery and Parent-Child Narratives* (pp. 92–105). Oxford: Oxford University Press.

Weisz, J. R., & Kazdin, A. E. (Eds.). (2017). *Evidence-Based Psychotherapies for Children and Adolescents* (3rd ed.). New York: Guilford.

Chapter 3

Object-relations theory in child development and in childhood play

FELT is built strongly upon the foundations of Object-relations theory. In FELT, Object-relations are best understood as an exchange of emotional and/ or psychological content between a Self and an Object. Thus, there are three parts to FELT Object-relations: 1) the Self, 2) the Object, and 3) what is going on between them. We will focus on each, independently, below, and then, later in the chapter, will explore how Object-relations manifest in childhood play, followed by an introduction to how therapists may respond to Object-relations in therapeutic play.

The Self

It is widely appreciated that a person's sense of self is a complex psychological process involving cognitive, social, and developmental themes, all of which interact to determine the general organization and construction of the Self (Harter, 2012). The topic of the Self is also rooted in rich history of psychological theory and research, dating as far back as the late 1800s and most prominently emerging with the writings of William James and his distinction between the "I"-self and the "Me"-self (James, 1890). The "I"-self was (and still is today) the active part of the Self, the *knower*, or the one who actually observes what is happening to/in the Self and the world around it. The "Me"-self, on the other hand, is the part of the Self that is being observed by the "I"-self. It is the object or product of all the things one knows about the Self and the world. James further elaborated that one could have multiple "Me"-selves, as constructed in different contexts and different social arenas. So, while the "I" remained constant, the "Me" adapted to the world around it, displaying different aspects of the Self to accommodate environmental needs. The Me that I project at work is different from the Me I project at home, which is different from the Me I project at social gatherings, or when I'm teaching, versus acting as a therapist. Similarly, the Me that I project with one client may be different from the Me I display with another, depending on the client's individual needs.

What is paramount, then, in being able to resolve in a healthy manner all the diverse "Me's" that one projects into the world is having an "I" that can

DOI: 10.4324/9781032693187-4

successfully integrate complex information into a meaningful whole. This requires an "I" that is able to see not only all the "Me's" of the Self, but also all the "Me's" of the rest of the environment (of everyone else who is around) too. Additionally, the "I" must also have enough power to control the "Me" that presents at different times, to optimally fit the environment. All of this is an extremely complex process that occurs, in most of us, most of the time, outside of conscious awareness. Further, not all "I's" are created equally. Some have an "I"-self that exerts too much control; some "I"-selves control too little. In fact, there are a number of disorders associated with a pathological "I"-self. The most striking example of a pathological "I"-self is Dissociative Identity Disorder (DID), formerly known as Multiple Personality Disorder. One of the reasons this disorder is so striking is because of its oddity, which has led to a lay fascination with the disorder, one that is commonly depicted in Hollywood films, in often disturbing (dramatized) ways. Still, DID is defined by the existence of multiple, unintegrated personalities, each of which usually takes on unique (and sometimes mystifying) characteristics that are different from the *host*, which is the term used to identify the personality that most often presents itself in a person with DID (though it may not be the "original" personality). To many who do not study advanced psychology and psychiatry, DID seems like a problem of having too many personalities. However, in reality, the problem is a lack of one – specifically, a person with DID can be said to lack the "I"-self, or, at least, the "I" is not fully operating. Without an overarching "I" to integrate all the "Me's" into a meaningful whole, the "Me's" become compartmentalized and run rampant. Thus is the importance of a functioning "I"-self.

DID is not the only disorder associated with a dysfunctional "I"-self. Several personality disorders are also well-associated with disturbances of identity. Borderline Personality Disorder (BPD) is well-known for this. In fact, one of the diagnostic criteria for BPD in the *DSM-5* is "identity disturbance: [a] markedly and persistently unstable self-image or sense of self" (American Psychiatric Association, 2013, p. 663). Furthermore, BPD can also include dissociative symptoms (i.e., problems with memory, spacing or blacking out), especially in the face of stress. Narcissistic Personality Disorder (NPD) is similar. In most patients with NPD, narcissistic symptoms can be seen as a paradoxical "cover" for an extremely fragile sense of self. In other words, to conceal a very fragile self, people with NPD will instead project a narcissistic self. The narcissistic self is not a true self, then, but rather a false self, meant to hide the interior fragility.

There are also less severe, but still potentially pathological, problems of the "I"-self. In childhood, for example, it is common for adolescents to develop mild distress at feeling "fake," when they present different selves in different scenarios. In this case, the "I" is suffering from normative developmental immaturity of childhood, rather than from a true pathology. In other words, adolescents, up until about age 18, on average, are not supposed to be able to integrate all the diverse "Me's" into a meaningful "I." Rather, the "I" is still in development and still figuring out how to manage the complexities of a multifaceted world. Similarly, it can be argued that any person who experiences a significant amount of variability in the world will be more challenged to develop their "I." In some ways, that's a good thing. Diversity ultimately breeds a more mature "I," but, the "I" must remain open-minded enough to adapt to that diversity. If not, a person can experience distress. This is the part of normative "I" development, then, that can be potentially pathological. The "I" needs more support when exposed to new things to be able to adapt properly. Without support and mentorship, the Self may not be able to adapt, and a person may then struggle more. It's during childhood, prior to maturity, that the "I" is most amenable to healthy growth. As the saying goes, it is far more difficult to shape hardened clay. Luckily, though, even hardened clay can be softened again under the right circumstances.

So, as noted just above, developing an "I" that functions as an accurate observer and adaptive actor is a tremendously high-maturity service, one that not all humans obtain naturally and that requires a combination of hard work and necessary conditions for survival. To be an effective therapist, one needs to have achieved a reasonably solid level of maturity in their own "I" development, because effective therapy requires a professional who can observe and modulate how their own identity interacts with, and (then hopefully) transforms for the better, the Self of the patient. Similarly, a patient who benefits from FELT does so directly through access to their "I"-self and through its ability to modulate their own internal emotional states. In other words, helping children develop a healthy "I"-self – one that functions within healthy normative developmental expectations – is a key treatment target for FELT. This is an important distinction, influenced by the psychoanalytic roots of FELT. Even though FELT in its current state was developed as a treatment for anxiety, anxiety is not actually the primary treatment target. Rather, **the primary treatment targets are healthy Object-relations through a healthy Self, healthy Object-representations, and healthy exchanges between the Self and Objects.**

To fully appreciate the healthy development of an "I"-self, it helps also to understand theories about self-determination, self-actualization, and the hierarchy of needs (Maslow, 1943). These theories postulate that a person cannot realize their true, actualized self without first meeting some baseline needs/conditions. Specifically, a person must experience themselves as being physically safe and having satisfied physiological needs (hunger, thirst, rest, warmth, etc.) before they can meet their psychological needs (i.e., for belongingness, love, esteem, etc.). Finally, if all else is met, one can achieve self-actualization, which is the peak at which one reaches their full potential. Maslow's hierarchy of needs has broad applications across all of human psychology, including psychotherapy. More explicitly, psychotherapy focused on developing an optimized, healthy Self cannot succeed if a person's lower-order needs are not first resolved. So FELT, being a therapy designed to bolster healthy Self and Object-relations, will often fail if lower-order needs (safety, security, physiology) are not first established. Still, the goal of FELT is not self-actualization. No child will reach self-actualization; it is developmentally impossible. Rather, the goal is to resolve psychological needs according to development. This goal will come into play more concretely in the case conceptualization section of this manual (see Chapter 6), but it is essential for therapists and professionals who wish to utilize FELT to understand how the Self develops across childhood. Only then can FELT be applied properly.

Postmodern views of the Self

If we fast forward about 100 years from James, we progress to a more postmodern view of the Self, with theories dominated by Gergen (1991), Lifton (1993), and Cushman (1995). These theorists, and others like them, have latched on to James' concept of the multiple "Me"-selves and applied it to modern society. What these theorists have observed is that in modern society (and even more so today than in the early 1990s) humans have become increasingly inundated with social connections, both real and imagined (more on this later). This "saturation" of the Self, as Gergen called it, requires that we constantly construct our sense of Self based on external definitions – what our environment predicates – and very rarely, if ever, do we as humans have the opportunity to observe the isolated, unified Self. In Self theory, the unified Self is often judged to be the gold standard of optimal psychological health. That is, to function at our healthiest, humans need to experience the various "Me"-selves as a unified whole, integrated by an all-seeing "I." Like the eye of Providence,[1] the "all-seeing I" functions, ideally, to provide oversight and meaning to the different "Me"-selves that are presented to the world. In this way, the "I"-self is not just a conscious observer, but an entity designed to unify and give meaning to the rest of our existence. The "I" guides us and, in some ways, serves as a lighthouse to steer a rogue "Me" back home, to keep the different "Me's" from losing their path back to unity.

Gergen, then, has argued that along with easy air travel, internet access, cell phones, and (if his book were written again today) social media, humans have become so saturated with social linkages that we now lack the ability to unify so many "Me"-selves into a meaningful whole. Instead, we are prone to the development of multiphrenia and an inharmonious discordance of multiple selves. Consequently, this lack of Self-unity translates to disorganized mental health, which subsequently manifests in increased amplitude and frequency of mental health concerns and disorders.

Similar to Gergen, Lifton (1993) wrote about the "protean self," named after the Greek god Proteus, who, in order to escape capture by humans who wished to consult his wisdom (for he was omniscient), could (and regularly would) assume the shape of any other creature/being. It is from this chameleon characteristic, in fact, that the term "protean" derived its modern English use – meaning "changeable in shape and form." So, Lifton's concept of the protean self captures this same idea. In this case, the protean self acts just like the god Proteus, changing the Self to avoid "capture" by the "I"-self. Consequently, the "I" cannot then account for what each protean "Me" needs to "say," and is flummoxed in its efforts to achieve unity. The protean self, then, is a constantly changing self. Lifton would say there is a version of the protean self that can be healthy – a sign of "resilience in fragmented times," as the subtitle of his book suggests. However, scholars also note that the protean self, like Gergen's saturated Self, increases vulnerability to fragmentation and disharmony.

As a consequence of disharmony, the Self in postmodern theory, then, is often relayed as the "empty self" (see Cushman, 1995) – a Self who has no real, concrete idea about who they really are. However, not all modern theorists are so pessimistic about the Self. Although we must all acknowledge that an overabundance of "Me-selves" can challenge the "I" to unify the whole, we must also agree that humans still possess a natural psychological pull, a *need* even, to establish an integrated Self. Psychologically, humans, when pressed, will almost always attempt to explain their actions within the context of a formed or forming Self-identity. If asked to do so, humans invariably are able to describe a core set of traits or personality characteristics that define who they believe they are. Of course, there will be variance and discrepancy in whether those Self-perceived traits match with objective reality and whether those Self-perceived traits always accurately predict behavior (they do not), but, psychologically, humans at least make an effort to describe themselves in broad, all-encompassing terms. These Self-representations are equally vital to our human psyche, and, importantly, they play a key role in daily decision making, especially in adulthood. They also represent a clear presence of an "I"-self, even if, at times, that "I" is not always able to fully reconcile every "Me."

Self-representations and traits: how we use words to define the Self

In our human efforts to describe the Self, we are able, when pressed, to generate identifying features that make us who we are. The work of Susan Harter (2012) is perhaps the most extensive review of this subject and how it occurs across the lifespan. Harter has researched the development of the Self for decades and has found interesting trends across different stages of development. Young children (ages 2–4), for example, when describing the Self tend toward concrete observable characteristics ("I have brown hair." "I have blue eyes.") and simple attributes focused on abilities, activities, possessions, and preferences ("I am fast." "I like spaghetti." "I love my dog."). These early Self-representations are rarely cohesive and often unrealistic. Young children go reliably through a stage of normal narcissism too, where they exaggerate their own abilities and conflate the actual Self with the ideal Self. So, even if a child is not actually a very fast runner, they may say, quite confidently, that they are, in fact, fast – blazingly fast, even. They may say things like, "Watch me throw this football! I bet I can throw it across the whole yard." Or, "I am perfect at ballet." Sometimes, they even make us parents feel great by directing that normal narcissism at us: "My dad cooks the best eggs in the world!" "My mom is stronger than Superman!" All of this is normal though, having no correlation with problems of the Self later in life.

Out of the normal narcissism characteristic of very early childhood, toddlers and preschoolers will typically approach the world with immense confidence, especially when they feel otherwise safe (i.e., if they know a caring adult is nearby to provide supervision). They will often display exhibitionistic-type behaviors – "Hey! Watch me do this awesome thing!" They are curious and strive for independence, while simultaneously longing to maintain a connection with caregivers. Separation anxiety is thus normal, maintained by a healthy awareness that the world is bigger and scarier than children are competent to handle alone. Still, separation anxiety should be neither too long-standing nor too intense. If such significant separation anxiety occurs, it can represent a lack of confidence in the Self to tolerate and face normal childhood stressors, a notable deviation from the "norm." On the other hand, confident independence does not mean outright rejection of caregiver assistance (although children may reject help in certain situations). Children should not be so confident that they abandon all caution and flee from caregiver boundaries. Instead, a healthy, confident, independent child is one who believes in their ideas and is active in trying to execute those ideas, but checks with and responds to others who limit risk with proper boundaries. This back-and-forth interaction can be seen when observing children in nearly any setting where a known adult caregiver is present. A healthy, confident child will explore a new environment somewhat freely, but only after seeking permission from the parent/caregiver. This permission-seeking may be more subtle in some than others, ranging from simply looking around to see if the caregiver is still present to cautiously standing by the parents' sides until sufficient "comfort" is achieved. Still, in healthy children, such behaviors occur eventually and reliably.

Following from the above, healthy children should also display at least some confidence, in reaction to stress, that soothing and recovery will eventually occur. They may become distressed in the face of stressors, and some may even become wildly distressed. But, in their distress, a healthy child is one who does *something* to relieve that stress. In some cases, that "something" may be an active form of self-soothing – sucking their thumb, hugging a stuffed animal, actively seeking an adult for comfort; in other cases, children may engage in more passive attempts to attain soothing – crying while waiting for an adult to come to them, calling for a parent (but not coming to them), etc. All of these are within the normal range of behaviors a child may display when stressed. An abnormal reaction to stress occurs when a child reliably does *nothing* in response to stress. Such a reaction is very rare, but in these cases, children appear indifferent to stressors, a form of learned helplessness,[2] where stressors seem inevitable and thus pointless to avoid. Learned helplessness, in turn, leads often to depression. More commonly, children still *try* to do something in response to stress, but they may become disorganized in their attempts, or become too easily frustrated and "give up" when faced with a challenge, or show developmental regression. These children are both incompetent *and* unconfident when facing challenges, an especially problematic combination.

Interestingly, a very young child's competence in handling problems is far less important than their confidence. Many children with the highest levels of confidence are some of the most incompetent, and vice versa. There are also many skilled children who lack confidence in their own skills. Still, the more important goal, at this preschool age, to developing a healthy Self is confidence. Competence can come later.

In early to middle childhood (ages 5–7), children usually are beginning school and as a result growing increasingly exposed to other children their age. As a result, they become a bit more realistic in their Self-appraisals (though they still aren't entirely accurate), comparing themselves to their peers and to their past selves. So, children this age still tend toward grossly positive Self-appraisals, but they are more selective about what they are good at, focusing on specific competencies. They tend to say things like, "I am getting faster as I get older." Or, "I'm still fast, but my friend Jill is faster." Or, "I once ate seven pancakes in one sitting!" In this stage, children also become increasingly able to internalize others' standard for regulation of behavior. In this way, a form of a "cultural self" (Nelson, 2003) begins to emerge. Now, the child's autobiographical self is shaped alongside a cultural framework, as prescribed by a culture's norms, standards, and values. This feature is especially salient in forming gender roles, which are particularly prominent in early childhood. Children this age tend to align with stereotypical gender roles as predicted within the greater culture. These gender identities may or may not conform with the gender assigned at birth. In most cases, incongruence between assigned gender and identified gender *traits* at this age does not translate necessarily to later transgender identity (de Vries & Cohen-Kettenis, 2012). More often, they are normal childhood explorations of the Self in relation to cultural norms. Parents in this stage can respond to identity explorations with openness, but they may also offer some kind editorial shaping to help the child figure out what fits them best. For example, as children notice their bodies and personalities changing over time, parents can help them recognize they are still the same person – "You may not be as fast as Jill, but you're still you, and I love *you*." Such commentary helps engender Self-continuity. Parents may also regulate excessive behaviors – "I remember when you ate seven pancakes, and you didn't feel so good afterward! Maybe this time we won't eat so many!" These interactions are important for building Self-regulation in children. Lastly, parents can breed positive self-esteem through unconditional positive regard – "Some boys like things that girls like and some girls like things that boys like, and that is okay. I love you no matter what you like."

Children in early to middle childhood also begin to develop an enhanced ability to "map" representations of the self and others onto one another (Fischer, 1980). Especially prominent at this age is the ability to link *opposites* in the mind. So, whereas very young children tend to believe that everyone is good at everything (universal positivity), older children reason that if one can be good at something, one can also be bad at something. This leads them to map their own Self-representations into a form of all-or-none thinking, where if someone is good at something, they are always good at it, and if they are bad at something, they are always bad at it. Similarly, if a child loves something, they always love it, and if they hate something, they always hate it. This leads to generalizations. If a young child eats broccoli once and hates it, they can become unwilling to try it again, no matter how differently their parents cook it. Or, if they have a favorite TV show, they fall in love with every episode, no matter how "bad" some episodes of the show might be. This all-or-none thinking can help protect social relationships in a way. Young children that have a conflict with a friend move on from it quickly, because they like their friend, and if they like their friend, they always like them, even if they aren't doing very likeable things. Of course, this also has a potentially dangerous downside. A child who is being harmed or abused by someone they like may not understand that what is happening is something "bad," because why would someone they like do something bad? Fortunately, children can learn that certain behaviors are bad, and this can help them reconcile that good people can do bad things, and can lead them to "tell on" others when they do bad things (even if they do like that person). Although sometimes this feature can turn a child into a "tattle tale," it also ensures they will tend to follow rules without questioning them. In their all-or-none thinking, young children see rules and morals as being absolute, without [really] questioning them.

Still, at this age, children also develop a capacity for understanding that others do not share the same mind as them (Theory of Mind), and thus, they can think and do things outside of others' awareness. This means that children will try to "get away" with breaking the rules at times. This occurs because children (and all humans in general, for that matter) are far more reward-focused than punishment-focused. If given a choice between seeking a reward or avoiding punishment, most children will choose the reward. So, if they think they can sneak a cookie without being caught, they will try to do so, because the reward of the cookie outweighs the threat of being caught. Parents can circumvent these behaviors by reinforcing compliance with rules/ expectations with rewards equal in salience to the rewards the child may get by breaking the rule. In this manner, children can learn that compliance is rewarding in and of itself, and perhaps even more rewarding than satisfying selfish, hedonistic desires.

Still, because children do now possess the theory of mind necessary to know their parents (and others) don't automatically know everything that goes on in their head, they are also now capable of projecting a "false self" into the world. Thus, it is at this stage that children show the first signs of a false self – that is, a self that is expressed to achieve a certain goal and is inconsistent with the true, or dominant self. However, some scholars disagree on whether there really is such a thing as a "false self." Some argue that all selves are true selves, that each self is capable of the spectrum of behaviors. So a "shy" person may be typically shy, so much so that shyness becomes a part of the identity, but that shy person may, in a pinch, push their limits and put on an "outgoing" mask (perhaps, for example, to impress a boss who values sociability in the workplace). Some would suggest this outgoing display is a "false self," whereas others may suggest it simply reflects that even shy people can be sociable in certain situations. In other words, rather than establishing a true versus false self, the person broadens their definition of the true self to include one who is capable of previously incongruent behaviors. This latter reasoning is the one I prefer personally, because it allows for a more nuanced view of the Self that is amenable to growth. This is especially important in psychotherapy, because it suggests that a person who has developed pathologi-cal aspects of the Self – e.g., "I am depressed," "I am a worrier" – is not "trapped" with that identity forever and can entertain and internalize healthier contrasts into the overall identity – "I am a person who sometimes gets depressed, but who chooses to fight it," or, "I worry, but I also have this part of me that wants to just let things go and be free." By practicing healthy coping skills, they are not projecting a "false" self. They are not "faking it until they make it." They are actively growing the former Self into a healthier being.

This same process is happening in children who project different selves in different situations. If you ask most children, "Are you a liar?" most will say, "No." If you ask them if they've ever told a lie though, most will answer honestly and say they have. This is even true of young children in this 5–7 age range. Their global Self-appraisal is positive – "I'm not a liar" – but they can, at times, tell lies, which does, technically, make them a liar after all. By being challenged with scenarios in which they choose to lie, yet still considering themselves not to be liars, they are pushed to consider that perhaps they can lie after all, which means that everyone can lie, which means that maybe even Mom and Dad are liars too. Most children will take several years to reconcile these ideas and realize that all humans are liars (capable of lying). It will take even longer before these same children are able to differentiate between what it means to be a liar (sometimes) and to be a liar by trait. As children move into adolescence and young adulthood, they learn that some people lie more than others, and that some people lie so much that they become untrust-worthy. When presented with these examples, they must build new cognitive schemata that allow for nuanced, individual variation and must develop an internal system that draws a line somewhere between behavior and trait.

The line between behavior and trait is an advanced concept that the Self typically does not finalize until adolescence and young adulthood, and different people draw that line at different points in the spectrum of behaviors. As an example, I've always felt the "fool me once, shame on you; fool me twice, shame on me" idiom to be overly harsh – certainly I can allow someone to make more than one mistake before I place them into the category of "bad." Others, though, are more cautious about to whom they offer their trust. They may actually draw a hard line at one mistake and blame themselves for not pushing others away who cross that line, saying, "I should've known better." Such differences are usually built upon a lifetime of experiences, where those who have been repeatedly hurt or taken advantage of by others are more likely to draw harder lines in their assessment of behavior versus trait, in an effort to protect the Self. Young children tend to be the most forgiving in this aspect; they can allow for great variability in behavior before they "assign" people to categorical traits. As reviewed above, some of this "forgivingness" is attributable to cognitive limitations in their ability to organize their thoughts about the Self and Others. Other reasons for infantile purity are that they are not changed by experience. As the Self is faced with an increasing number of Objects in the world, it must develop an organizational system for these Objects. Categorizing others based on traits, rather than behaviors, allows for a more efficient cognitive organizational system. If everyone lies, the behavior of lying doesn't separate one person from another. But if some people who lie a lot can be called "Liars," then developing an internalized "folder" in the mind for Liars helps people assess their world more efficiently. So, one key feature of the development of trait language is enough experience with enough people/ Objects that it becomes necessary to build neural "folders" and filters through which to view the world. Children usually will not reach that level of experience until late childhood (9–11 years).

One important job of child psychotherapy is to catch children when they are young enough and help them build, as early as possible, a Self that is neither hyper- nor hyposensitive to categorization of Objects. The real world is complex, and real Objects defy categorization. It is not psychologically healthy, then, to "assign" traits to people based on limited information. However, we know that children who experience early, chronic trauma (especially interpersonal trauma) tend to do just that. Thus, intense and/or prolonged, unusually negative experiences will prime a person to develop a method to rapidly assess the safety of their world. It is a survival mechanism designed to protect the integrity of the body and the Self. Such children will tend toward categorization of others based on limited information. For some, if an adult seems friendly and likeable, they will attach to them somewhat indiscriminately, seeking a relational connection with anyone willing to give it to them. Others may instead become so cautious they resist attachment, and when opportunities for attachment present themselves, they may act in a dis-organized, but vicious way to push the Object away, or at least to them know, "Don't mess with me! If you want this relationship, you better be serious about it!" These behaviors happen because these traumatized children have developed a schema that tells them either that "adults will love me if I show them affection" or that "adults might hurt me, even if they seem to love me." Both indicate a hypo- and hypersensitivity to relational attachment and both reflect a confusion about the differences between traits and behaviors.

Traumatic experiences can also affect Self-representations. In the above examples, the indiscriminately attached child develops a Self as one that is loved based on his or her actions. In the reactively non-attached child, the Self is one that is unworthy of love, no matter what they do. Both cases are considerable aberrations from the natural healthy Self that is prototypical of young children – the overly positive, competent Self. So, even at this young age, adverse experiences can grossly affect the Self, and the examples given here are only two extreme examples. There are other possibilities. A depressed child may view the Self as boring. An anxious Self may lack specific compe-tencies. A hyperactive Self may be plagued by chronic loss of control.

Importantly, although children in early to middle childhood are capable of describing the Self, they tend to show low interest in scrutinizing the Self. The "I"-self is active, able to observe and describe the "Me"-selves, but it does not yet possess the metacognition necessary to also observe and evaluate the "I"-self itself. So, the I can describe the Me, but not the I. In the above examples, a traumatized, anxious, depressed, or hyperactive six-year-old will struggle immensely to analyze how those emotional states – those "Me's" – interact with the Self-identity. They can tell you they feel unloved, scared, sad, or out of control, but the internal processes that drive these states will escape them. Furthermore, a young child will show no real interest in even trying to describe the "I"-self. Such advanced metacognition usually does not take place until at least adolescence, though it can emerge in late childhood. Nonetheless, **children can benefit from a therapist's examinations of the child's "I"-self**. Thus, if a therapist spots an "I"-self in a child that fails to accurately moderate the whole environment, the therapist may then work to build the child's overall gestalt of the Self. For example, in play, a child may take on the role of rescuer, playing the hero in a way that suggests they are exploring the heroic aspects of their own Self, their pull to care for others, protect others, and solve problems. In doing so, the child may ignore the complex impact such caregiving has on the hero-self, and the therapist may then wish to invite the child to explore this concept, perhaps suggesting, "Whew! I bet Captain America is tired after all that rescuing!" or, "I bet sometimes Spiderman wishes he could take a rest from being the hero." Through these playful interactions, therapists can help children connect with parts of the Self through the therapist's analytic skills, knowing that the child's own skills are not developed enough to address such complex content on their own.

As children progress toward middle to late childhood (8–11 years old), they show many of the same aspects of the Self as their slightly younger counterparts, but with a bit more self-coherence, agency, self-efficacy, and self-continuity. Abilities that just emerged in early childhood now mature, but don't yet solidify (solidification of the Self comes much later). Peer pressures also begin to pick up and further influence the cultural self. Children at this age may start self-criticism, as influenced, in part, by cultural norms. They may wish to look or dress different. They may express despair that they aren't as good at sports as they once believed. They learn that not everyone automatically likes them, and they don't automatically like everyone either. Thus, they may start to form subgroups in their social circle – a better-identified "friend group" – rather than simply being "friends" with everyone in their class. They may also express a desire to be "popular." In learning that others may not like them, they can start to become self-conscious about how they present in different social circles.

In middle to late childhood, emotional maturity also grows. They build a more robust emotional language, and they become more sophisticated in being able to express that one can *be* happy, but still experience sadness, or worry, or any other emotion at the same time. Thus, children move away from all-or-nothing thinking and instead toward a more nuanced appraisal of the Self and of Others. This nuance allows them to form and build a more accurate Object-relational framework, but it also makes the world a bit more confusing and scary. Suddenly, instead of blissful ignorance, children are thinking more deeply about how the world works, from which predictably emerge heightened fears and worries. In fact, middle to late childhood is the time in which children are expected to normatively peak in their fears and worries (Muris, Merkelbach, & Collaris, 1997; Ollendick & King, 1991). So, even if children consider their world to be a generally safe place, they recognize that bad things can still happen. They may develop nighttime fears no longer focused on being afraid of the dark or monsters under the bed, but they worry about realistic (albeit catastrophic, and unlikely) threats like a home invasion, or a storm destroying their house, or their family going to sleep and not waking back up. They may worry if friends will still like them after a summer vacation and will care more deeply about small details in their appearance, no longer pleased with a "good enough" gestalt. It is not that as younger children they did not *notice* details; in fact, children of all ages pick up on far more in their environment than most adults give them credit for. Instead, older children both notice *and think about the implications of* details. As a result, anxiety can take hold, drawing the child's thoughts toward negative implications/outcomes, over positive ones.

Since FELT is not expected to be applied to children beyond late childhood, an exploration of Self-development during adolescence and early adulthood is beyond the scope of this manual.

Therapeutic goals that derive from vulnerabilities of the Self across childhood

The features of the Self as defined in this chapter not only outline how the Self changes over time; they also guide therapists and other professionals about the targets of healthy Self-development. Because of these developmental phases of the Self, children can encounter specific vulnerabilities of the Self at different ages as well. Protecting children from vulnerability to pathology of the Self, then, is key to the FELT paradigm. As stated throughout this manual, FELT itself is not designed to respond to symptoms alone. It is designed to direct healthy development of Object-relations, which requires, as a baseline, assisting children to build the healthiest Self possible at each given developmental stage.

Therapeutic goals for Self-development at different ages applicable for FELT are outlined below.

Goals for Self-development in very early childhood (ages 2–4)

Given what we know about the normal presentation of the Self in healthy preschool children, we can now set concrete goals for Self-development. Pediatric therapists working with preschool-aged children should set goals to inflate the Self, which is often achieved through consistent, repetitive positive feedback from multiple caregivers. When a preschooler engages in exhibitionistic behavior, they are offered the rapt attention of an audience who seeks only to build them up. Therapists can encourage this attention without worrying that doing so will overinflate self-esteem or breed long-term narcissism. Rather, such self-aggrandizing exchanges are essential to healthy development in young children.

Pediatric therapists should also work to build confidence in preschoolers, giving them space and freedom to explore their environment and their ideas, while encouraging supervision from adults. Therapists intervene to build an environment in which responsible adults do provide routine oversight and boundaries, but who are not so overbearing as to never allow children to explore their independence. When children do become distressed by the big, scary world, therapists can also help them develop healthy soothing skills, which should involve a combination of self-soothing as well as a recognition that adults are there to help when help is needed.

Lastly, therapists can work with preschoolers to develop a rudimentary Self-narrative, where they are able to describe the Self in developmentally appropriate terms. If there is evidence of an impoverished Self (inability to describe the Self – what they like, what they want, what makes them "them"), therapists help to correct this by aiding children to discover themselves. Therapists can achieve this through modeling, revealing a bit about themselves in the process, but within a proper developmental lens ("I have brown

Table 3.1 Norms and abnormalities of Self-development from ages 2 to 11

Age range	Norms of the Self	Abnormalities/Deviations from norms	Therapeutic goals
2–4 years	Defined by simple attributes, observable characteristics, and possessions Normal narcissism/inflated Self Incoherent Self All-or-none thinking	Negative Self Lack of exhibitionistic play Lack of confidence in own ideas and/or abilities Extreme reactivity to change or stress No reactivity (ever) to change or stress Impoverished Self (lack of narrative about the Self)	Inflate the Self through consistent, repetitive positive feedback Encourage healthy exhibitionism Encourage healthy reliance on adult caregivers Build self-soothing skills Develop a primitive narrative of the Self
5–7 years	Defined by specific competencies More elaborate attributes (more complex) All-or-none thinking (though less pronounced than previously) Able to link opposites Generally positive view of Self, but more accurate Compares Self to Others and to past Self Increased knowledge about the "standards" of society (but lacks integration of society into the Self)	Grossly negative Self (no/low recognition of strengths) Grossly positive Self (no recognition of weaknesses) Overly egocentric – unable to consider Others' points of view Ignorance of the past Self Ignorance of societal standards	Build a nuanced Self – recognizes strengths and weaknesses Promote optimistic view of the Self's potential for growth Build awareness of Others Build the Self-narrative, recognizing changes in the Self over time
8–11 years	Trait labels, including specific abilities and personality characteristics Compares the Self to peers More integrative, balanced thinking (not all-or-nothing) Increased accuracy of Self-appraisals Societal standards guide the Self	Grossly negative or positive views of the Self Excessive egocentrism Fails to understand how Self-descriptions fit with societal norms All-or-nothing thinking persists	Build a nuanced Self, with accurate appraisals of strengths and weaknesses Balance past Self with new Self Balance societal norms with existing personality traits, and vice versa

hair." "I love pizza." "I have two brothers."). They can also help by observing what describes the child – "You have blue eyes." "You really like a lot of action in your play." "You're a great talker." They then wait for the child to respond, perhaps correcting or shaping observations to the child's own observations of the Self.

Goals for Self-development in early to middle childhood (ages 5–7)

As children move toward early elementary ages, pediatric therapists shift focus away from deliberate overinflation of the child's Self toward a more nuanced Self, one that recognizes individual strengths and weaknesses. Therapists can use coached interviewing to promote children this age thinking in more complex ways about the Self. They may say, "A lot of kids have things they're great at, and then things they are not so good at. What about you?" Modeling also works here – "When I was young, I was good at math, but not so good at sports." The very reasons children come to therapy can also be used to stimulate discussion about weaknesses – "One of the reasons we meet together is because sometimes you get really scared and don't know how to feel better." Throughout these discussions, therapists work to promote more accuracy in the child's overview of the Self, but children do not need to be completely accurate. They may continue to say they are great at math, even if they are really only average, and such positive appraisals are in fact healthy for them.

As weaknesses are discussed, the therapist works also to promote an optimistic view about the child's potential for growth. Again, this can be done in discussing reasons for therapy: "You might be a worrier, but I can help you learn how not to let your worry control your whole life." Therapists can also encourage parents to recognize how the child has changed over time. Parents can show the child baby pictures and note, "Look how much you've grown." They can then reflect on skills or traits the child has developed over time. These examples highlight for the child that growth and change are possible. At this age, though, therapists refrain from in-depth co-analysis (with the child) about *how* growth or change has occurred, as these children are not interested in that analysis. They may be able to describe new skills that occurred during the change, and they may even connect those new skills to changes in the Self – "I used to be bad at reading, but once I started practicing everyday I got better, and now I'm pretty good at it." However, diving into exactly what happened during reading (e.g., improving phonics, fluidity, comprehension, etc.) is typically beyond the capacity or need of children at this age. This same metaphor applies to growth from mental health complaints.

Therapists can also help early elementary children by building their awareness of Others. I often test a child's baseline ability to describe Others by having them tell me about their friends. At this age, children most often will name their friends and (when prompted) what things they like to do with them. As they move further into middle childhood, they may be able to elaborate specifically what they like in a friend (e.g., they are funny, kind, like the same things). Children this age are unlikely to describe how they behave or act differently around different peers, and they are unlikely to express strong preferences for specific "types" of playmates (girls versus boys; older kids versus younger kids). But, these children should at least have some emerging awareness that people have individual differences among them and should be able to describe ways they are different from Others (and vice versa) when prompted. Children who lack this ability to notice individual differences can build this ability in therapy. FELT achieves this through play and by structuring play in such a way as to highlight individual differences and how those differences shape a character's experience of the play.

Goals for Self-development in middle to late childhood (ages 8–11)

At this final stage of childhood to which FELT is applied, therapists work to continue to build a more nuanced Self, increasing the accuracy of a child's appraisals of the Self and their strengths and weaknesses. In later elementary years, children typically have begun to connect with more specific peer groups, and they may also have separated themselves from other peers with whom they do not connect closely. It is rare in this separation that a child this age says they "do not get along" with others. Rather, they remain friendly with peers outside their closest group, but they can acknowledge why connections with some peers are easier than others. Usually, peer groups are formed based on complementary strengths and weaknesses. So, children with similar strengths or interests tend to match together. Children this age rarely "branch out" for the sake of branching out. They instead stick to what they like or to things very close to what they like. Thus, children who have not found a "fit" in a friend group or who still have not identified specific "likes" and interests may need assistance from therapists to find their "place" in their environment. Therapists can help such children find interests by building skills in trying new things. They should also be prepared to address specific barriers, such as social or performance anxiety, poverty, or logistics, that may interfere with the ability to try specific interests. For this reason, it is often useful for therapists to be aware of and connected to various other child-interest groups in their communities, which may include sports leagues, scouts, YMCA, art institutes/classes, crafting, and other extracurricular activities kids may want to try outside of school. They should also work to build familiarity with social service organizations that help families who cannot afford to do so, or who have other logistic boundaries, to participate in these activities.

By late childhood, kids should be able to reflect more deeply on the Self and how it fits with their immediate environment. They can describe rudimentary social norms and how those norms dictate their own behaviors. They can also reflect upon the past Self and how it fits with the newer, more "current" Self. Therapists can help children who struggle with these connections by focusing play and other therapeutic interventions on building inter- and intra-personal reflective capacity. So, a play intervention might be created in which there are characters that represent the child and others in the child's life. Therapists then watch how the child plays with and labels these characters, with an eye toward moving the child toward accurate labeling of intra- and inter-personal processes taking place during the play. More specifics of these play interventions are outlined in Part II of this book.

Objects

In Object-relations theory, an "Object" is any thing with which the Self builds a relationship. Objects can include people, animals, things, places, etc. They can also include both real and imagined Objects and real and imagined relationships. Primary Objects represent those Objects for which we create a direct internal representation inside our psyche. Secondary Objects represent those that are internalized because they connect to or remind us of a primary Object. Tertiary Objects remind of secondary Objects, quaternary of tertiary, and so on. Classically, the main historical focus on Objects in Object-relations theory was on real people present in a person's life or history. Other Objects (animals, things, places) were argued to be important only because of their connection with real people. For example, the most well-known and commonly used secondary Objects include the pacifier and other comfort Objects (blankie, stuffed animal, etc.), which often become important to children not so much because of their inherent value but because they replace the comfort and nurturing normally offered by a parent when that parent is not around or otherwise unavailable. In such cases, secondary Objects help fill a gap when primary Objects are insufficient. Just because they are secondary (or tertiary, or quaternary, or so on) does not make "replacement" Objects less important or have less value. In fact, a person's attachment to a secondary Object can become quite pronounced, perhaps even, in some cases, more pronounced than their attachment to the primary Object. This is especially true if the primary Object itself has unsafe, unattractive, or other undesirable properties. In such cases, a secondary Object can take on the idealized version of the primary Object, such that the secondary Object more reliably comes through, even when the primary one fails. If the primary Object then makes frequent, egregious failures, the secondary Object can start to take on characteristics that better fulfill the psychological needs of the Self. When this happens, secondary Objects can transition toward primacy.

Take the following example. Sarah is an eight-year-old female who lives with her mother alone as an only child. She does not know her father at all. Mother struggles with severe recurrent depression, which at times leaves her with flat, unresponsive emotion and anhedonia (lack of enjoyment) for daily activities, including caring for Sarah's emotional needs. Sarah also has a stuffed pig that her mother got for her when she was younger, during a time when mother was not depressed and more her normal self. During mother's depressive episodes, Sarah uses the pig to help remind her of her mother when she was at her best. The pig, then, takes on all the best qualities of her mother. Over time, the longer mother's depression lasts, the more Sarah comes to rely on the pig to fulfill her needs for nurturing and love. Sarah may even begin to forget that the pig is a representation of mother and begins to see the pig as a mother-like figure itself. As this happens, the pig begins to transition into a primary Object in Sarah's life, where she relies almost exclusively on her pig to provide for her psychological and emotional needs, realizing that mother is no longer capable of doing so.

Though the above example is heartbreaking when it occurs in real life, it highlights two important features of childhood psychology that are worth noting here. First, children can be extremely resilient in the face of hardship. In Sarah's case, even though her mother struggled with severe mental illness, she developed a way to cope, even in her young age, and to meet her own needs when mother was unable. Second, it reveals the potential healing power of replacement Objects. *Replacement Objects, in fact, can be the difference between pathology and wellness.* This feature of Object-relations theory is particularly important in the underlying mechanisms of change employed through FELT. Throughout treatment, FELT uses play to build healthy secondary Objects and resolve unmet psychological needs that drive pathology. The unmet needs that drive pathology are described in more detail in Chapter 4, but for now, the important message is that resolving unmet Object-relational needs is a core treatment target of FELT.

Internal representations of Objects

In the Object-relations theory used in FELT, our *internal representations* of Objects matter far more than the actual Objects themselves. For example, Sarah's mother in the example above may, in actuality, be doing a relatively poor job of mothering during her depressive episodes. This is not to say that she is a bad mother – she is ill and needs help; I only mean that objectively Sarah's mother fails, when depressed, to meet her daughter's needs. This happens at some level to all parents. We are all, as parents, imperfect, and we do a lot wrong in our journey of parenthood. Our imperfections do not make us bad parents. On the contrary, they make us normal. Donald Winnicott (1953), a founding father of modern attachment and Object-relations theory, wrote extensively and beautifully about the concept of "good enough mothering," which specifically highlights the fact that healthy children do not need perfect parents and, in fact, benefit in some ways from parenting failures. He wrote that the mothers' failures to adapt to every need of their children help them adapt to external realities (Winnicott, 1953). In other words, Winnicott taught us that a "good enough" Object is one that adapts its physical and emotional attunement according to the individual developmental needs of each child at different stages of maturation. A good enough Object does *not* provide every need at all times, but rather challenges the child to build increasing levels of Self-control and relative independence from the Object.

Still, what matters most is the *internal representation* of the Object as being "good enough." A mature, healthy Object-relation is one in which the Self (specifically the "I"-Self) realizes that no one is perfect and that real people are nuanced and complicated. By matching internal representations with the complexities of real people, a person is able to relate better with their world, with the people in it, and, in fact, with themselves. Thus, it is partially through the influence of "good enough" Objects that one is able to refrain from splitting Objects into extreme versions and, subsequently, from also splitting the Self.

Splitting occurs when a complex Object, with both good and bad qualities, becomes split, psychologically, into two or more different internal representations. Splitting is an unhealthy adaptation designed to simplify the world to make it more predictable. If a person splits Objects into specific categories, they can then better predict behavior based on those categorical representations. A loving person will do loving things. A selfish person will do selfish things. A neglectful person will neglect. A punisher will punish. A giver will give. In reality, all people are capable of loving, of selfishness, of neglect, of punishing, and of giving, and ideally, a goal of Object-relations is for us to develop internal representations that reflect that reality. But, splitting is simpler and, many times, safer, protecting a person from psychological and emotional harm at being "let down" by imperfect Objects. People not only split Objects, but, as discussed previously in reviewing theories of the Self, can split the Self. An unintegrated, fragmented, disharmonic Self is a split Self, but it is through relating at early ages to imperfect Objects, and then not resolving the internal psychological conflict created by complex imperfections, that a person develops that pathological adaptation of splitting, pushing them to then split the Self as well.

So, splitting Objects breeds splitting the Self, and both actions create vulnerabilities to mental illness. Just like it is better to integrate the Self, it is also better to integrate Objects. Returning to our example of Sarah, Sarah will increase her chances of resilience by internalizing all parts of her mother as a meaningful whole. Yes, mother is, at times, sad, withdrawn, unavailable, and maybe even irritable, but mother is also loving, nurturing, selfless, and generous. If Sarah can hold onto those "good" parts of her mother, even while realizing she also has some "bad" qualities, she can, perhaps, internalize mother as being "good enough," which protects her from splitting. If, on the other hand, Sarah copes by splitting, she may identify two different internal representations of "mother" – one that is loving, nurturing, selfless, and generous and another that is sad, withdrawn, unavailable, and irritable. Such splitting can cause an incredible amount of confusion and paradoxical reactions later in life when Object-relations are activated by other forces. Of course, Sarah, being a small child, has little to no conscious control over whether or not she integrates or splits her complex mother. Rather, a child's internalized representations of Objects tend to be shaped by those of their caregivers. A mother who splits the Self and splits Others is likely to generate those same tendencies in her children, simply through subtle (or at times not so subtle) communications over the child's life about Object-relations. Similarly, a child who receives well-integrated messages about others is also likely to build well-integrated messages themselves.

Healthy Object-relations are nuanced and can be quite object-specific. A person with optimal Object-relations may develop an internalized representation of their own mother, but they are able to differentiate this relation from other mothers they may encounter in life. They can separate their own mother from other mothers. Unhealthy Object-relations, on the other hand, tend to be overgeneralized and infiltrate numerous relationships. As such, an unhealthy Object-relation can be triggered by extraneous stimuli, which can, in turn, have detrimental effects on the Self and on the person's relationships with new Objects. In the split Sarah above, we have a split mother Object – one good, and one bad. Because unhealthy Object-relations predict generalizations, split Sarah would be prone, throughout life, to experience all relationships that trigger the Object-relation in a predictable way. That is, if she encounters a strict teacher, one who is perhaps well-meaning, but who has acquired a reputation of being tough, demanding, and perhaps less forgiving than other teachers, Sarah's interactions with this teacher may trigger the "bad mother" Object in her internalized representations. She may then form extremely negative reactions to this teacher, who is now split into the "bad mother" Object, without also having the "good mother" side to balance it out. This teacher then becomes the enemy, and a nasty cycle may ensue, a sort of self-fulfilling prophecy where Sarah believes she can do nothing to please the teacher, and so she either stops trying, or she tries extra hard, only to feel disappointed when she eventually misses the mark. In both cases, the unconscious act of sorting this teacher internally into the "bad mother Object" category can become a significant source of distress for Sarah, which in turn activates the Self that Sarah has attached to that "bad mother" Object. In this case, Sarah's Self in relation to the "bad mother" may be one that is inadequate and disappointing. If the bad mother Object is triggered by external reminders, Sarah is then prone herself to feel suddenly inadequate and disappointing again. This can occur even if the actual bad mother – that is, Sarah's real mother who was originally split into her good and bad parts – has not actually done anything (this time) to activate the bad mother Object. Instead, it was triggered by this strict teacher, and Sarah's internal psychology couldn't tell the difference.

A key goal of Object-relations psychotherapy, then, is to help clients integrate Objects, rather than split them, and to improve differentiation between different Objects. Through differentiation, the "teacher" is no longer confused with the "bad mother." Instead, the child/client is challenged to consider 1) that the object (the teacher) is its own unique Object (differentiation); 2) that the Object has some good parts, in addition to bad parts (integration); 3) that the child's Self has value without regard to how they have been treated in the past (Self-differentiation); and 4) that the child themself also has good and bad parts (Self-integration). The latter two goals were covered previously in the section on the Self. We will cover the former two in more detail below.

Object differentiation

Object differentiation refers to the separation of internal representations in one's psyche. Humans have a natural cognitive tendency toward sorting and grouping. Categorization facilitates memory structure and allows us to access linked concepts more easily from a mental standpoint, and we do it with pretty much everything. We have broad mental categories, such as animals, plants, colors, things you can eat, furniture, etc. From broad categories, we can create refined subcategories. Under animals, for example, we can further specify mammals, birds, reptiles, amphibians, and so on. More advanced levels of knowledge allow for even further/more complex refinements. So, biologists and zoologists can name *chordate* animals and animals within the *Panthera* genus. Similarly, many botanists can recognize different species of *Hibiscus*. Special scientific knowledge also allows those same botanists to name the properties that make each species fit into the *Hibiscus* genus and to specify how the *Hibiscus* differs from a similar, but different genus, *Hibiscadelphus*. [3] However, without sufficient knowledge, differentiation becomes difficult. Sure, we can all differentiate between animals and plants, mammals and birds, and so on, but the general public usually will not know whether the cheetah is in the *Panthera* genus (it is not; the cheetah has its own genus, *Acinonyx*) unless they've been specifically and credibly taught that information.

Differentiation of internal representations follows a similar trajectory. In our natural movement toward categorization, humans want to group other humans together into sensical categories. We do this in both simple and complex ways. As noted previously in the section describing Self-development over time, young children tend to categorize Others first by their physical characteristics. There are boys, girls, White people, Black people, tall people, and short people. As we age and as we build more knowledge, we can make more refined classifications – people who are kind, people who are mean, people who like art, people who like sports. We can also begin to see the overlap in these categorizations. We understand that it is possible for a person to like both art and sports. We may even create a whole third category to accommodate this overlap. So, we have a group for people who only like art, one for those who only like sports, and one for those who like both. Increased knowledge and maturity also allow people to understand that some categories are not absolute. For example, a person who is 6'3" is tall in most circumstances, but in the NBA, rather short. So, a person can be simultaneously tall and short, depending on the context. A person who is mixed race – let's say White and Black – may be "dark skinned" when around a bunch of Caucasians but may be "light skinned" when compared to someone with two parents of African descent. So, maturity and knowledge allow us to boost the complexity of categorizations of Others. By educating children (at proper developmental levels) about healthy, nuanced Objects, pediatric caregivers, including therapists, can help create a structure for children to develop their own healthy Object-relations. But doing so is not always easy.

Internal representations of personality and psychology are extremely complex, far more difficult to categorize than physical characteristics or personal preferences above. What makes them so complex is that behavior is not easily predictable from personality. Just because someone is "dependable" doesn't mean they will literally always come through on others' expectations of them. Similarly, a "hard-worker" is likely to have some moments of "laziness" too. For this reason, it is not practical to form impressions of someone's personality based on a small sample of behaviors. If we catch them on an "off day," our first impression of someone may not be representative of who they usually are. Further, even if first impressions are accurate, they are never complete. To fully understand another person, we have to spend a lot of time with them.

Unfortunately though, spending a lot of time with people comes with great risk. If we don't really know who someone is, how can we be sure they are even safe to be around? This is especially hard if we've had people in our past who have hurt us after we've taken the risk of trying to get to know them. For this reason, it can be extremely difficult for someone with a history of adverse relational experiences to build the necessary knowledge to promote healthy Object differentiation. If they've been hurt before, and they are cautious to get close to people to avoid being hurt again, then they can never get to know people well enough to challenge the predispositions/broad categorizations. Instead, it is safer to just assume that everyone can hurt you and then to set up barriers to minimize the harm. This is why it is so hard to repair Object splitting, especially later in life. Splitting is a defense to minimize harm, and asking someone to challenge that splitting is asking them to put themselves at risk again of more harm.

Still, the goal of therapeutic Object differentiation is to repair the effects of Object splitting. First, it is important to note that though the terminology is similar, splitting and differentiation refer to separate behaviors. Remember, splitting involves taking a single, complex individual and splitting their psyche/personality into multiple parts, as a means to simplify their categorization. To return to Sarah and her mother, Sarah split her mother into good and bad because this helps her better predict which mother she is going to get at any time. When good mother is around, she can relax; when bad mother is around, she must be alert and ready for anything. So, splitting is an unhealthy psychological action to defend against unpredictable changes in a single person and to try to make that person more predictable. Differentiation, however, is a healthy psychological action designed to understand that not all other Objects are necessarily the same. The reason splitting is unhealthy is that it *significantly* increases a person's risk of engaging in indifferentiation, in which all Objects are essentially treated equally, and indifferentiation is a poor strategy because it does not reflect reality. People *are* different and should be treated differently.[4]

To return to our previous botany metaphor, differentiation can mean the difference between life and death sometimes. The morel mushroom is a highly sought-after, edible mushroom common to the USA. The false morel, on the other hand, looks very similar to the true morel, but is actually quite poisonous and potentially deadly. Knowing this, many with an untrained eye are taught from an early age to avoid eating all wild mushrooms, to avoid making fatal mistakes. This is an example of indifferentiation. Someone with proper training, however, can learn to easily identify differences between true morels and false morels. With diligence, they can take steps to make sure mistakes are never made and they never mistakenly consume the morel's poisonous cousin. In this case, adequate knowledge helped them overcome indifferentiation.

Humans can learn to do the same with our internal representations. With proper training, even early-ingrained fears of Others caused by indifferentiation can be unlearned, and people can learn to trust Others again. Now, this process/training is not as easy as learning how to identify a true morel, because, as described above, human personality is more complex and less predictable than are the physical characteristics of mushrooms. Still, a major therapeutic goal of FELT is to determine a child's relative levels of Object differentiation, determine if those levels are unhealthy for their age, and then act to help that differentiation move in healthier directions as needed. This process is typically completed through a combination of Play Therapy – using play objects to help teach differentiation inside therapy – and parent coaching – teaching parents how to communicate with their children at home to reinforce healthy Object differentiation. The specific techniques through which this goal is accomplished are outlined in Part II of this book.

Object integration

Object integration has much overlap with Object differentiation, in that indifferentiation is often a predictable outcome of a failure in Object integration and they both derive from similar life experiences. Object integration involves the specific understanding that individuals do simultaneously possess both good and bad (or, more accurately, acceptable and unacceptable) traits. Integration is a psychologically mature skill that usually does not present reliably until middle childhood, though some children show evidence of the skill in early childhood. Splitting is the opposite of Object integration.

Splitting is considered a psychological vulnerability, but, unlike Object indifferentiation, splitting does not always lead to grossly unhealthy outcomes. Consider the stage of normal childhood, for example, where a young boy splits his image of father, such that only the "good/acceptable" parts are entered into the child's internal representation of father (and the "bad" parts are just ignored or denied). In early childhood, this stage of "hero worship" for parents or for other important people in a child's life is considered protective. It is seen in healthy children around the world and is widely accepted by mental health professionals as being a characteristic that improves a child's chances of healthy psychological development later in life. It is also a form of splitting. So, splitting is not always undesirable. Still, splitting is a primitive defense that only works if there is relatively little need for psychological defenses in the first place. In other words, it works well in children who form secure attachments with securely attached caregivers, and only early in life, when dependence needs override needs for autonomy and Self-development. Later in life, though, when dependence needs must contend with at least equally important needs for autonomy and other needs of the Self, splitting becomes an unsatisfactory defense.

Splitting stops working because, at some point, the human mind must contend with the fact that the Self and Others are intricately related. In order for one to understand themselves, they must understand Others, and vice versa. In infancy and very early childhood, most children do not need to understand the Self very deeply. It is enough to just understand Others, and only at a rudimentary level – will this person take care of my needs as a dependent on them? If Others do provide sufficient care, infants and very young children can get by ignoring the "bad parts" of these caregivers. It's like, "If you're keeping me alive, I guess I can overlook the fact that sometimes you get frustrated with me." It's when the child develops other needs – those not focused exclusively on dependence – that splitting becomes no longer tenable. As reviewed in the previous section on Self development, as children age, their Self-needs become increasingly complex, and splitting can't accommodate those complex needs for long. So, when splitting continues past the dependency stage of development, it creates psychological vulnerabilities that breed an array of unhealthy functioning/symptoms. This is because splitting does require a denial of reality. In reality, people are complex and have good and bad parts, and so splitting requires a continued distortion of reality. Furthermore, humans understand the Self through understanding Others. So, by splitting Objects, humans also split the Self, and a split Self (which will be described in more detail below) creates split emotions, split behaviors, and more split relationships.

Object integration, then, is an essential goal for optimizing all healthy human development. Object integration can only result when several basic core factors are present first. Safety is paramount. A child who cannot establish a sense of safety cannot resolve the dependent stage of development, and thus they cannot adequately prepare themselves to move beyond the natural, healthy splitting stage and into Object integration. Risks to a child's safety include a multitude of stressors and adverse childhood experiences (ACEs), including, but not limited to, trauma, poverty, caregiver separations, severe illness, unresolved grief, and other stressors. As referenced above, Object integration also requires relative maturity. Young children are *expected* to engage in at least some splitting, and even if their external demonstrations suggest an understanding that humans can be both "good" and "bad," their internal representations are usually split, and usually toward the positive. So, we know from clinical and developmental research and observation that Object integration requires maturity. This fact pushes researchers then to ask ourselves why? What are the cognitive maturations that are necessary for Object integration?

As of the date of this book, I am unable to locate specific research that has identified the cognitive components necessary to build a capacity for Object integration. Still, we can make some educated guesses based on what we do know about child development. First, children must develop a capacity to psychologically separate the Self from Others. Margaret Mahler[5] (Mahler & Furer, 1968) wrote extensively about several important concepts in describing how children relate to Others over the lifespan. Mahler originally proposed a stage she named *normal autism*, which described the first two to four weeks of a child's life when they seemed relatively unaware, psychologically, that Others exist. In its original form, normal autism, then, defined the idea that there is a time when children seem to be so completely focused on the Self that they are unaware of external stimuli unless those stimuli also affect the Self. In other words, for a newborn infant, if the infant is not experiencing something in the moment, that thing does not exist, *and*, importantly, the infant cannot do anything to manipulate the environment to bring that thing into existence. During normal autism, then, infants are just reacting to what is around them, and they do not understand that they can actually act to affect their world.

Infants learn pretty quickly, though, that if they cry, someone will usually come to help them. This stimulates the emergence of the *normal symbiosis* stage of Mahler's theory. During normal symbiosis, infants can now understand that they coexist with Others in their world, and that in such coexistence each person can affect the other – baby affects parent, parent affects baby. This stage lasts about five to six months until the separation-individuation stage starts. During separation-individuation, the child finally understands that they exist *independently* from Others. The earliest signs of this stage usually involve separation anxiety, where the child has now realized that "if I can exist independently, then I can be alone, and I don't like that." Separation-individuation continues for a long time (the rest of the child's life, in fact), growing increasingly complex and changing in manifestation over time, with the child growing more comfortable as they age with increased separations from caregivers. Still, in order to reach Object integration, a child *must* first enter the separation-individuation stage; in particular, they must also progress to the late version of this stage, called "Object constancy," which refers to the final concept that Objects, and their properties, generally do not change.

Object constancy, as I use the term here, encompasses a wide variety of skills/cognitive understandings allowing children to maintain internalized representations of Objects. Object permanence is one of the earliest-emerging and best-known examples of Object constancy. Piaget (1957) originally described Object permanence as occurring at the end of his sensorimotor stage of child development (which lasts from birth to about two years of age). Classically, Object permanence has been documented by a child's attempts to search for an Object after it has been hidden from sight, and whether they search for that Object in its understood hiding spot. For example, if a toy is covered with a blanket, a child with Object permanence will look under the blanket for that toy. Updated research has amended Piaget's theory and has explored Object permanence at earlier stages (as early as three to six months) (Moore & Meltzoff, 1999). This newer research has found that even though very young children do not engage in a motor act to search for a missing toy or missing Object, they do show increased interest in stimuli that test Object permanence (meaning they do *notice* that something "weird" has happened). So, there are interesting signs that Object permanence occurs much earlier than we previously believed.

Another well-known example of Object constancy also comes from Piaget's research and can be seen in the cognitive ability of "conservation." Conservation is often tested through conservation of liquid. In the classic experiment, children are shown two (or more) different containers of water, each container of a different size. Taller containers will appear fuller than shorter, wider containers, even if they have the same amount of liquid in them. Typically, children understand conservation and will report that the amount of liquid remains the same regardless of which container it's in somewhere between ages 7 and 12 (Piaget, 1965). Conservation, then, is a more advanced version of Object constancy where children begin to understand that properties of Objects can change without actually changing the Object (i.e., "The water appears to be less in this container, even though I know that it's still the same volume of water.").

Now, if we apply these abilities to our psychological understanding of other humans, we can see similar trajectories. Very young children (infants) can understand that just because Mom or Dad are not in the room, they do not literally cease to exist (Object permanence). However, they may cry if Dad suddenly shaves his beard, not quite recognizing that he's the same person (a failure of conservation). Over time, though, children become more and more capable of adapting their internal representations. Eventually, they can see that Dad is still Dad – beard or not – because the beard does not define the dad. This realization – that Dad doesn't need a beard to still be Dad – is an early sign of Object integration, that Dad is a sum of his parts, and that taking away one part does not make all the other parts cease to be. As children learn more about what does, in fact, make Dad "Dad," they must integrate more parts to make sense of Dad. Furthermore, if Dad does something out of character, something that doesn't "fit in" with the current image of Dad, the child must then decide if this new behavior can just be ignored or discarded or if it also has to be integrated into a new image of "Dad." A good example of this is when kids begin to realize that their parents have psychological flaws. For example, they may find when Dad is tired and hungry, he gets grumpy, and they should not push his buttons during that time. This may not be a behavior, then, that they ignore. In fact, this characteristic becomes important to integrate into the new image, as it means they should watch for signs that Dad may not be in a mood for nonsense. On the other hand, if a dad who is usually attentive, loving, and involved one day forgets to attend his son's baseball game (for which he apologizes), this might be a behavior that can be ignored as an anomaly, chucked from the child's memory as an irrelevant mistake that doesn't change who Dad really is.

It's experiences like these that shape a child's internal representations, and they happen constantly. Every new experience for a child in their Object-relations with a caregiver must either be integrated or ignored. However, sometimes integration fails. Integration failure usually occurs because an important behavior has happened reliably and the child does not have the psychological maturity or support to integrate that behavior into their conceptualization of the caregiver. So, let's say this dad who is otherwise attentive and loving misses multiple baseball games, and let's say he eventually stops apologizing and reconciling with his son after these missed games. Now, the son gets confused, "How can my Dad who loves me not care about my games?" This confusion, if not resolved, can eventually cause the son to split Dad. On the one hand, Dad loves me. On the other, Dad isn't present. This is just one of infinite examples of how splitting starts. So, another requirement for healthy Object integration is for children to have healthy supports to guide them through confusing incongruities in their Object-relations. Most children do get these supports from parents, teachers, friends, and others – people who are there to show/tell them that "No one is perfect," or that "Sometimes a parent won't always be there with you in person, but they are still with you 'in spirit.'" These lessons serve to help children stabilize Object-relations through integration. Thus, it is important in psychotherapy to ensure children get these supportive lessons to help move them toward Object integration.

The final proposed necessary component for children to develop Object integration is that they need genuinely "good enough" role models. "Good enough" internal representations were reviewed previously in this chapter. They are highlighted again here to help demonstrate their specific importance in Object integration. If an Object, in reality, is not genuinely "good enough," that is, if they actually fail in their role often enough to fall short of the "good enough" bar, that Object probably will not be well-integrated. This occurs because, psychologically, the child still internalizes archetypes of what different Objects should be. A mother or father is supposed to be loving, nurturing, and attentive. A teacher is supposed to demonstrate genuine care for the education of others. A police officer is supposed to "serve and protect." When a child's real-life experiences do not fit with these archetypes though, they will still split Objects internally between the archetypal representation and the experienced representation. In other words, a child who suffers from caregiving that doesn't meet the "good enough" standard (perhaps a parent is abusive and neglectful for many years) may develop internalized representations of a "bad parent." Even though that "bad parent" internalization is not entirely inaccurate, the child can still recognize – especially as they get older – that it does not match with the archetypal expectation of what a parent is supposed to be. This realization is then what causes a split parent Object, in this case.

Another negative consequence can occur from a failure to integrate archetypal internalizations with experienced internalizations. After enough experiences incongruent with the archetype, a person can begin to change the archetype itself. A relevant example of this occurs in attitudes toward police officers in the USA. In the USA, different individuals carry different beliefs about the archetype of police officers. For some citizens, police still hold the classic "serve and protect" archetype. They are seen as heroes who sacrifice their potential safety in service of others. For other citizens, police are seen as abusive tyrants, with a purpose of oppressing others through force and intimidation. In this case, there is a split archetype, then. Some people are able to integrate the split archetype – some officers are "good," *and* some are "bad." Those who can integrate can maintain that both conditions can be simultaneously true. Those who cannot integrate split the archetype.

Again, this splitting creates a psychological vulnerability because it does not reflect reality. In reality, it *is* definitely true that some police officers are good and some are bad. This is true of any profession, really. It's also true that on occasion bad cops can be known to do good things (e.g., arrest real, dangerous criminals) and good cops can be known to do bad/unethical things (e.g., letting someone out of a traffic ticket as a "personal favor"). So, splitting the archetype and splitting individual cops both require a distortion of reality. The distortions can create a vulnerability because they can easily lead an individual to be distrustful of police. Consequently, that individual may not reach out to police when they have a problem for which police could be helpful. Furthermore, if they face a police officer, they may become exceedingly anxious, which in turn can cause the officer to become suspicious. This is especially true if the officer themself also has split archetypes about our person in this example. Let's say, for example, that the person in this story is a member of a minority group who get arrested at higher rates in the USA

(Gase et al., 2016). In this case, the police officer may develop a prejudice – that is, a split archetype – for the minority group, which in turn predisposes them toward suspicion that a person of that minority group is more likely to break the law than others.

Now, we end up with a dangerous mix of two people who are interacting with each other through split archetypes, which can cause neither to perceive the other accurately. An officer who is genuinely offering help is seen as a predator who can cause significant harm, and the person needing help is seen as someone who is probably up to no good. Unfortunately, we have recently seen far too often what happens in these situations. This is one of the reasons we need police reform in the USA – we need to fix the split archetypes present and move them toward Object integration. In my opinion, police reform starts when we fill the streets with enough "good enough" officers that the ones who are not "good enough" have minimal to no effect on the archetype.

This same principle applies to children who have split any other archetype – mother, teacher, doctor, etc. Children have to be presented with real evidence of sufficient "good enough" examples of these archetypes before they can ever form healthy, integrated archetypes. To know a "good enough" mother, they have to see, over and over again, good enough mothering. To trust teachers, they need to see most of their teachers are "good enough." Therapists must keep this in mind on multiple levels. To boost a child's Object integration, therapists need to 1) work to support that child's real caregivers – parents, other family, teachers, etc. – to be "good enough"; 2) present/project play-based representations of "good enough" Objects widely and profusely; and 3) be alert to and intervene accordingly when a child engages in splitting beyond the developmentally normative stage.

In sum, Object integration requires four essential components:

1   Children must possess a cognitive ability to separate the Self from Others. In most children, this will happen automatically in very early childhood. However, some children fail to resolve this completely, and they continuously fail to truly separate the integrity of their Self-identity from internalized Object-representations (and clinically, people who never resolve these primitive needs create vulnerabilities to later developing personality disorders such as borderline, antagonistic, or dependent personality traits).

2   For full Object integration, children must progress to mature levels of Object constancy. Developmentally, completely matured Object constancy is not expected to occur until after late adolescence. So, for most children in therapy, the goal is not to reach completely matured Object constancy, but, rather, to facilitate the growth of Object constancy through supports and therapeutic feedback.

3   To reach full maturity, Object constancy needs reliable support throughout development. Children need regular reminders toward Object integration.

Therapists are advised to look for opportunities to reinforce these reminders in treatment and to teach caregivers how to reinforce them at home.

4   Children need genuinely "good enough" caregiving to accomplish Object and archetypal integrations. If they are in an abusive or otherwise insufficient caregiving situation, they are unlikely to achieve Object integration until that caregiving situation is remedied.

The "in-between" – the relationship between Self and Objects

In the beginning of this chapter, I introduced Object-relations as having three components: the Self, the Object, and what is happening between them. It is this third part that we come to now. Split Sarah may develop split selves in relation to each split mother Object. The "good" mother may trigger positive aspects of the Self – one who is loved, well-cared for, accepted, valued. Inside this relation between the loving mother and the beloved Self, Sarah may experience positive emotions like joy and warmth. She is comfortable receiving kindness from Others and seeks close relationships with Others. The "bad" mother, on the other hand, may trigger a "bad" Self. She may reason something like, "If my own mother is sad around me, ignores me, rejects me, or gets mad when I speak to her, then I must not be very valuable, or a disappointment, and I do everything wrong." If this becomes Sarah's Self-representation inside the "bad mother" Object-relation, she will then express that through negative emotions and behaviors consistent with the Object-relation – she will withdraw, become self-critical, and perhaps stop "trying," becoming apathetic. These behaviors are what I refer to as the "in-between." They are what we therapists (and others) can more easily observe – the overt manifestations of internal Object-relations.

Later in life, Sarah may encounter other figures that trigger the "mother" representation – teachers, therapists, friends, boyfriends, girlfriends, etc. Any person she meets in her life that shows any qualities of the split mother Object may create confusion for Sarah, simultaneously activating both the "good" and the "bad" mother Objects inside Sarah's psyche. So, if a teacher is kind and nurturing toward her, Sarah may initially feel warmth and joy, but she may also feel paradoxically sad and withdrawn. She may not understand why she feels these negative emotions in response to a teacher being kind to her, but they are there, nonetheless. Similarly, Sarah may also find herself mysteriously drawn, perhaps as a teenager or in adulthood, toward relationships with other "bad" people. She may seek boyfriends or girlfriends who neglect her or are irritable toward her, because, despite these bad qualities, they also trigger for her the potential for good qualities. She is seeking her mother. Alternatively, she may build a personality that wants to care for those who are hurting or sad. This may be especially true if, in her original "bad mother" Object-relation, she took on a Self that became the parent/caretaker for her mother. Such an Object-relation predicts (though it does not guarantee) that Sarah may activate this part of her Self anytime the "bad mother" Object is triggered in her life.

The above discussion focused on "mother" Objects, but humans can presumably develop infinite numbers of internal representations about Objects in our lives. In fact, internal representations are commonly made for all the archetypes discussed previously in this chapter. Humans develop Object-relations for all of these archetypes, and each may contain various levels of wellness versus pathology. So, for example, a person may develop a healthy Object-relation for mother, but an unhealthy one for father. Alternatively, parents and close friends can be healthy, but teacher and ruler could be faulty. It is rather rare (though not impossible) for someone to have all Object-relations be completely healthy. An absence of any healthy Object-relations is often a cause of major and pervasive psychiatric disturbance. The most common Object-relations profile is one whose core Object-relations function relatively well, but peripheral archetypes may cause them some distress from time to time. Thus, though an ideal goal may be to develop globally healthy Object-relations, it can be good enough to aim for the core relations and then allow healthy core relations to also translate to healthy peripheral ones.

During the childhood phases in which FELT is applied (generally, ages 4–11, though these ages are not absolute), children are vulnerable to several predictable impacts of Object-relations. First, cognitively, young children naturally struggle with understanding that Objects can simultaneously possess attributes of opposing valence (e.g., good and bad, kind and mean, strong and weak). Some children can do this better than others, and based on my own clinical experience, I would argue that children in general are more capable of opposite-valence simultaneity than classic research seems to suggest. This difference of opinion is mainly due to variations in how cognitive abilities were assessed in the research studies that established this finding. Namely, classic research studies relied on expressive verbal ability, which is already limited in younger children. Though researchers have found creative workarounds to accommodate limited expressive ability, the research designs still do not permit a complete observation of how children express and understand complexity. Namely, as outlined in Chapter 1, children most naturally explore and express complexity through play. I have observed, through childhood play, in both clinical and research settings, a tremendous ability for even very young children to display complex characters with both positive and negative qualities simultaneously. Thus, even though asking children about attributes generally produces one-sided views of others (which are, most times, overwhelmingly positive), observing their spontaneous creative play reveals more complex appreciations of human personality, including what seems to be at least a basic understanding that most humans can be both "good" and "bad" at the same time. Thus, if we observe childhood play, we can see that children can, *in fact*, understand complex, opposite-valence attributes in Objects around them, even if they do not verbalize their understanding in as concrete a way as a more mature brain would.

Still, one challenge for young children is to *concretize* complex Object-relations in a meaningful way. Although they can intuitively understand that humans are complex creatures with multifaceted "Me's," they are cognitively limited in their ability to allow abstract realities to direct and influence behavior. Experience and age both shape the application of cognitive abilities; that is why a 34-year-old with an IQ of 130 can accomplish far more than a 4-year-old with a 130 IQ. Cognitive ability only goes so far. Thus, although cognitively children *can* understand complex Object-relations, their young age and lack of experience limit how much complexity they can hold in mind at any given time, and, perhaps more importantly, limit what they actually do with that baseline ability.

A further limitation is that in humans across the lifespan, Object-relations rarely cross the barrier into consciousness. For most of us, Object-relations exist and influence behavior in our unconscious minds. Even in the mature mind, Object-relations operate outside of awareness, and it is only when we make a purposeful effort to do so that we can bring our Object-relations forward into conscious awareness. To be able to do so, one must be able to engage in introspection and must have the ego strength[6] to tolerate endeavors into the unconscious with honesty, integrity, and an objective, analytic mindset. Both research and clinical experience tell us that even adults are typically incapable of a perfectly honest, objective view of the Self, and the many threats to one's ego strength include stress (both chronic and acute), genetics, and development. Now, genetics, it should be noted, give a more indirect influence on ego strength, in a similar manner to how genetics influence any aspect of personality, a review of which is beyond this scope of this book. For now, it suffices to know simply that ego strength is neither constant nor unlimited. It can be developed or damaged through life experiences, but theoretically can only grow within a certain range (similar to IQ). It is well known that a person inherits IQ within a *reaction range,* such that a person with both parents and most immediate blood relatives with IQs in the 70s is extremely unlikely to have an IQ of 150. They may achieve, especially with enrichment, an IQ well above their parents (e.g., in the 100s), but their genetics will limit their growth in IQ. On the other hand, IQ can be much more easily damaged than enhanced. Brain damage, malnutrition, severe neglect, or other insults can severely lower IQ. Similarly, a child who is the progeny of relatively low ego strength is unlikely to max out the scale of ego strength, even if that child gets the best support in the world for building ego strength. They may surpass their parents, but it certainly won't come as easily to them as to a person who inherited superb ego strength. Also, just like IQ can be more easily damaged than developed, a person's ego strength can also be severely inhibited by life events.

So, as we are examining a client's ability to use their Object-relations, we must consider their relative ego strength not just with regard to their current ability but also with regard to what is the potential of their ego strength.

Children, by virtue of their age and immaturity, should not be expected to reach the ego strength, at least while still young, of a fully matured adult. As such, they should neither be expected to engage in the kinds of introspective, objective analysis of Object-relations that an adult could do in practice. For that reason, Object-relations psychotherapy with children looks very different than its adult counterpart. The therapist's goal is **not** to help bring a child's Object-relations into conscious awareness, because most children are not expected to be capable of this. Rather, the goal is to shape the child's environment and enrich their growth in such a way as to allow optimal Object-relations to develop where possible and to repair Object-relations where necessary. All of this is done in the unconscious. So, a major challenge of FELT is that the therapist is constantly operating inside a child's unconscious.

To operate in someone else's unconscious requires 1) a tremendous amount of cautious responsibility and 2) a particularly strong ego that can manage multiple "I"-selves at the same time – namely, that of the therapist, of the client, and, at least part of the time, of parents too. Many of these therapist characteristics (and others) are reviewed in Chapter 5, and it is important for therapists who work in the unconscious to take a careful inventory of their own selves to ensure they are prepared to practice responsibly within the unconscious mind. Such preparation is no easy feat, requiring years of training and an ongoing mentality toward maintaining competence throughout one's career. However, when a clinician takes proper steps to prepare for the unconscious, they can work there to promote long-lasting, meaningful change in their clients.

The accuracy of internal representations

Importantly, internal representations can be wildly inaccurate at times. Because Object-relations are filtered both through Objects and through the Self, internal representations can be distorted at times by faults in the Self and by overgeneralization of Object-relations. A core tenet of FELT is that one cannot correct inaccurate internal representations without also correcting the filters. Other therapeutic approaches, like CBT, for example, do place a heavy focus on correcting inaccurate cognitive distortions about the world. And though CBT "purists" rarely describe the mechanism of change in CBT as directed at Object-relations, I do believe a change in Object-relations is one of the reasons CBT techniques are so effective. As people learn to challenge cognitive distortions about the Self, Others, and the world, they subsequently adjust their own Object-relations. In FELT terms, then, changing thoughts using CBT techniques is akin to changing an Object-relations filter in FELT. In FELT, once a person changes their filter, their sense of Self and Others (and consequently, their overall mental health) also changes. Thus, in practice and in methods, FELT shares quite a bit of overlap with other existing evidence-based treatments for childhood disorders (namely, CBT), just using different terminology and underlying goals.

Distortions of the Self can take many forms. As reviewed previously in this chapter, some distortions of the Self are transient and developmentally normative. For example, normal narcissism and overestimation of performance are characteristic of early childhood. Adolescence, on the other hand, is characterized by an overly egocentric Self, where teens commonly overvalue their own importance in their immediate world. The cognitive, developmental, and social sources of these normally phased distortions of Self are widely discussed in social and developmental psychology literature.

It's when distortions of the Self persist beyond developmentally normal phases that they can cause longer-term pathology. But how does one know when a self-image is inaccurate? If someone's "I"-self says they are a bad person, it will always be able to find evidence – even if distorted or biased evidence – that they are, in fact, a bad person. If a clinician trains that "I"-self to attend less on the evidence of "bad" and more on the evidence of "good," how do we know, then, that the clinician is accurate? After all, what if this client actually is "bad," and looking at the "good" is a mental distortion, rather than the other way around? In truth, this argument is one I have seen regularly in my work, especially with self-deprecating or depressed teens. They tell me, "You're only saying that because you're my therapist and you *have* to. But what if I'm really none of that (good stuff)." Honestly, these teens have a point. I cannot *prove* that they are, in fact, objectively "good." But focusing on accuracy often misses the point. Instead of arguing for *accurate* Self-representations, I find it easier to argue for *healthy* Self-representations. Healthy Self-representations, as reviewed previously, are integrated and differentiated. A healthy Self is able to recognize that it is simultaneously both good and bad, but that it has *choice* in how it uses that information to approach the world. **So, among a clinician's most pressing tasks in psychotherapy is to help clients develop the power of** *choice* **in how they use their Self-image to interact with the world around them.**

When we see "bad" internal representations, it is not always as important to replace the "bad" with "good." Rather, it is more important to challenge clients to accept that they have "bad" qualities – either inherently (as imperfect humans) or as a result of their experiences. From there, they can integrate those qualities into a more meaningful whole. They do not have to split themselves into good and bad. They can be both, and they can choose behaviors that most consistently fit with the Self they want to be. From there, clinicians must also help clients identify a balanced, healthy Self to work toward. This is why it is so important for therapists to understand deeply what makes a healthy Self. Only then can we help clients imagine and reach that healthy Self themselves.

Real versus imagined relationships and their impact on Object-relations

Another important topic of exploration in this chapter has to do with what types of social relationships matter in our definition of the Self. In some of my own writings/research, developed in large part through collaboration with my very first graduate student, Dr. Michael Feeney, to whom I owe a great debt in being a sounding board and collaborator in building the following theories, I have described *proximal* and *distal* influences on the construction of the Self. These constructs capture the fact that humans use a combination of both real and "imagined" relationships to define the Self. Proximal relationships are defined as those in which there is or has been at some point a real, ongoing, reciprocal relationship between a Self and an Object. Common proximal influences include family, friends, teachers, mentors, coaches, etc. Distal influences, on the other hand, can occur when humans use non-reciprocal relationships to influence their identity. Common examples of distal influences include celebrities, historical figures, ancestors, and fictional characters. It is not uncommon for us humans to see role models in people we have never met and are never going to meet. For such relationships, we know about them (the Others), but they do not know about us. Still, the lack of reciprocity in relationships does not always mean they have less of an impact on our identity. We've all had a "hero" in our past that inspired us to change something about ourselves, without us ever even interacting with that person. For me, there was Michael Jordan, who made me want to be awesome at basketball (and other sports), and for a time that mattered a lot, though not anymore. There was Dr. Sean Maguire, the psychologist portrayed by Robin Williams in the film *Good Will Hunting*, who became my first inspiration to become a therapist (and that one still matters to me today). There are authors of books, articles, and theories that I read that make me think in new ways or teach me new skills that I use in everyday life. There are countless further examples. For most, we've found in our research, these distal relationships do not *replace* proximal relationships, but they do supplement them and play important roles in the process of forming Self-identities.

When learning and executing the lessons taught throughout this manual and throughout FELT, distal influences are regularly used through play scenes to help children develop healthier internal representations of the Self and Others. FELT therapists routinely model a wider variety of relational input – both through actual therapist/client relations (a proximal relationship) and through play-based representations of relations (distal relationships). By introducing children to a broad, healthy variety of relational modeling, and by then moving those Object-relations in healthier directions, the FELT therapist hopes to resolve psychological conflicts that predispose to psychiatric symptoms (see "Insight, re-experiencing, and working through," Chapter 4). This model, and the focus on directly altering in therapeutic ways a child's Object-relational framework, is what differentiates FELT from other evidence-based models for treating childhood anxiety and other psychiatric disorders. Most other evidence-based treatments for childhood disorders focus on symptom reduction through teaching coping skills and maintaining those coping skills long term. Such a method is efficient, practical, and often achieves, as a secondary goal, the establishment of healthier Object-relations and definitions of the Self. Thus, other established treatments are not at all "discredited" by FELT and should be readily used when useful in a clinician's toolbelt. However, in other treatments, developing a healthy Self-identity is a secondary outcome, more like a positive side-effect than a direct target of treatment. In FELT, building a healthy Object-relations framework is a primary treatment target, alongside and equal in importance to the goals of symptom reduction and building coping skills.

Notes

1   This metaphor of the "all-seeing I" is an allusion to the "all seeing eye" of Providence depicted in many religious and historical traditions. In such traditions, it is understood that there is an all-seeing eye of some supreme being, reflecting omniscience but also, in many traditions, benevolence and discipline. The all-seeing eye knows everything and works to unify a person's actions into a meaningful existence. It often forces humans to ask ourselves, "Is what I'm doing pleasing to divinity?"
2   In classic studies of learned helplessness (which would now be unethical), researchers administered an electric shock to dogs while "trapping" the dogs in a box which they could not escape. At first, the dogs showed distress and tried to escape the box, but over time, they eventually learned there was nothing they could do and they just lay down and took the shocks. This behavior continued even after researchers removed the "blocks" that were keeping the dogs inside the box. So, even when they could escape, they no longer tried, because they had already previously learned there was no point in trying. It was only after being shown again they could escape (i.e., being pushed outside the box) that dogs learned again they could actually get away from the electric shocks. Learned helplessness, then, can be unlearned.
3   Not being a botanist, I unfortunately cannot tell you the differences between these genera.
4   This statement does not adequately capture the nuances of equity, fairness, and universal human rights properly, which would be beyond the scope of this manual. It is true all people deserve fairness and equal access to opportunities, privileges, and basic rights. At the same time, I believe it is a great show of respect to treat people according to their individual needs and personality. In this way, treating people differently, if not otherwise violating their rights, can be a perfectly healthy way to communicate, "I see you, and I care about you enough to change my perspectives and behaviors to fit your needs."
5   Although Mahler's ideas are considered by many to be rather outdated in their terminology, I present them here for their historical context, while also explaining their utility in modern Object-relations theory.
6   For the reader unfamiliar with the term, *ego strength* refers to a person's psychological capacity to create balance between their hedonistic, self-serving, instinctual desires and interests (the *id*, in Freudian language) and their internalized, moralistic sense of right versus wrong (the *superego*). In fact, the original German for "ego" was "Ich" or "I." So, the ego is, for all intents and purposes, the "I"-self. The ideal ego is one that meets both needs of the id and the superego; ego strength is the ego's relative ability to satisfy both, which can vary over time and in reaction to life events (i.e., stress can decrease ego strength).

REFERENCES

American Psychiatric Association. (2013). *Diagnostic and Statistical Manual of Mental Disorders* (5th ed.). Washington, DC: American Psychiatric Publishing.

Cushman, P. (1995). *Constructing the Self, Constructing America: A Cultural History of Psychotherapy*. Boston, MA: Addison Wesley.

de Vries, A. L. C., & Cohen-Kettenis, P. T. (2012). Clinical management of gender dysphoria in children and adolescents: the Dutch Approach. *Journal of Homosexuality*, 59 (3), 301–320.

Fischer, K. W. (1980). A theory of cognitive development: the control and construction of hierarchies of skills. *Psychological Review*, 87(6), 477–531.

Gase, L. N., Glenn, B. A., Gomez, L. M., Kyo, T., Inkelas, M., & Ponce, N. A. (2016). Understanding racial and ethnic disparities in arrest: the role of individual, home, school, and community characteristics. *Race and Social Problems*, 8(4), 296–312.

Gergen, K. J. (1991). *The Saturated Self*. New York: Basic Books.

Harter, S. (2012). *The Construction of the Self: Developmental and Sociocultural Foundations* (2nd ed.). New York: Guilford.

James, W. (1890). *Principles of Psychology*. New York: Henry Holt and Co.

Lifton, R. J. (1993). *The Protean Self*. New York: Basic Books.

Mahler, M. S., & Furer, M. (1968). *On Human Symbiosis and the Vicissitudes of Individuation: I. Infantile Psychosis*. Madison, CT: International Universities Press.

Maslow, A. H. (1943). A theory of human motivation. *Psychological Review*, 50(4), 370–396.

Moore, M. K., & Meltzoff, A. N. (1999). New findings on object permanence: a developmental difference between two types of occlusion. *British Journal of Developmental Psychology*, 17(4), 623–644.

Muris, P., Merkelbach, H., & Collaris, R. (1997). Common childhood fears and their origins. *Behaviour Research and Therapy*, 35(10), 929–937.

Nelson, K. (2003). Narrative and self, myth, and memory: emergence of the cultural self. In R. Fivush & C. A. Haden (Eds.), *Autobiographical Memory and the Construction of a Narrative Self* (pp. 3–28). Mahwah, NJ: Erlbaum.

Ollendick, T. H., & King, N. J. (1991). Origins of childhood fears: an evaluation of Rachman's theory of fear acquisition. *Behaviour Research and Therapy*, 29(2), 117–123.

Piaget, J. (1957). *Construction of Reality in the Child*. London: Routledge & Kegan Paul.

Piaget, J. (1965). *The Child's Conception of Number*. New York: W. W. Norton.

Winnicott, D. W. (1953). Transitional objects and transitional phenomena: a study of the first not-me possession. *International Journal of Psychoanalysis*, 34(2), 89–97.

Chapter 4

Mechanisms of change in psychotherapy

How a therapist acts in psychotherapy depends significantly upon how one conceptualizes the specific mechanisms of change to be used in a therapeutic approach. In FELT, an integrative model of change influences not only the design of FELT but also how a therapist chooses, with each individual client, how they will implement various FELT interventions.

Sandra Russ (2004) outlined five[1] major mechanisms of change that occur in individual child therapy. In FELT, each of these is offered equal "footing" with regard to their potential to drive change in a child.

Expression, catharsis, and labeling of feelings

The first mechanism of change discussed here is also perhaps one of the oldest tenets of talk therapy. It is believed that through the simple expression of feelings, a child is able to *release* the emotional tension driving that emotion, which in turn resolves the emotion. Under this mechanism of change, it is enough just to "get a feeling out" for that release to be therapeutic. Theoretically, catharsis relies on the metaphor of a limited vessel of emotions. When this vessel is full, a child cannot function optimally, cannot respond in a healthy manner to their immediate environment, and tends to be driven too much by emotion, compared to other survival skills. By periodically emptying the vessel through catharsis, a child's emotional "battery" is recharged, and they can thus act more healthily.

Corrective emotional experience

In catharsis, it is enough simply to express an emotion and release. In the mechanistic theory of a corrective emotional experience, though, catharsis is only healthy if the release of emotion is perceived (by the Self) as being corrective, accepted, and contained. A wild, uncontrolled release of emotion, for example, can be very unhealthy, and can have potentially long-standing, detrimental ramifications. For some, punching your boss in the face when they make you angry may feel good (emotionally) for a moment, but if your boss

DOI: 10.4324/9781032693187-5

fires you or presses charges (or both), that uncontrolled release of emotion no longer served you. In fact, it may have made things worse. So, in order for a person to experience a corrective emotional experience, emotions need not necessarily be *released*, but, rather, they must be contained or managed. Therapists frequently serve as the containers or managers of a child's emotions, letting them release the emotions safely within the confines of a therapeutic relationship, where those emotions can be received, repackaged, and then returned to the child in a more manageable parcel. Such repackaging occurs partially through an Object-relational framework, with the therapist working to use healthy Objects (which can be the therapist, parents, toys, or anything) to shape a child's emotional reaction toward healthy expression.

Insight, re-experiencing, and working through

This third mechanism of change is also among the oldest in psychotherapeutic theory, originally derived directly from the theories of Freud and his acolytes (though with increasing nuance and complexity as theories have developed over the past century). This mechanism, then, is based on the assumption that humans (starting from childhood) have essential psychological needs that present early in life (within the first few years) and need to be resolved in a healthy manner in order to ward off psychopathology. There are a multitude of psychological needs outlined throughout the history of psychological literature. In FELT, though, we focus on seven primary psychodynamic needs which need resolution during childhood and throughout life.

1   A need to be free from pain/comfortable (analgesia/comfort needs)
2   A need to feel at least some level of power (*dunamis* and *exousia* [2] needs)
3   A need to meet one's own expectations for the Self (superego needs)
4   A need to be loved by Others, particularly a primary attachment figure (need for love)
5   A need for something to love (need for Objects)
6   A need to be well-liked and well-received by Others who are not attachment figures (popularity needs)
7   A need for a unified, true Self (integration needs)

Analgesia/comfort needs

Analgesia/comfort needs are believed to be the most primitive, presenting earliest in development, even before birth. For the purposes of this review, though, it is important to first establish that freedom from pain in this context does not necessarily always mean physical pain. Rather, it is more generalized and can indicate physical and psychological pain as well as all forms of discomforts. In this sense, humans naturally, all else being equal, will prefer comfort over pain. Even prenatal fetuses will avoid noxious stimuli beginning at the latest by 25–26 weeks of gestation (Craig et al., 1993). Neurobiological reactions to noxious stimuli can also be seen as early as 25–26 weeks of gestation (Slater et al., 2006).

Sure, there will be times in life when humans may choose to endure comfort or pain in order to accomplish a higher-order task, but usually these choices are made also in order for humans to avoid what is judged to be a greater pain. For example, we vaccinate to minimize risk of more serious illness. We endure exercise perhaps to prolong lifespan or to achieve that "rockin'" beach body physique, which may help provide social or self-esteem benefits. We study to accomplish academic goals and further our career. All of these behaviors are times in which we choose "work" over "play," because we've decided that working now is less of a "pain" than the alternative. The point is that both unconscious human instinct and reasoned life choices try to protect us from pain/discomfort.

When analgesic/comfort needs are unresolved, psychologically, humans will then tend to behave in ways designed to prioritize analgesia/comfort over other psychological needs, perhaps to their detriment. As with all of our core psychological needs, the key to healthy functioning is balance. No one should be completely free of pain and, as well, no one who is constantly in pain is likely to function optimally. It is just as unhealthy to seek to be constantly free of pain/discomfort as it is to constantly seek painful/uncomfortable things – though the latter may be harder to imagine (is anyone really, after all, unremittingly masochistic, always doing whatever hurts them most?).

There are key signs that may indicate a person/child is engaging in excessive avoidance of pain/discomfort. Most common, perhaps,[3] is a person who is unable to tolerate any discomfort for any reasonable amount of time. Such children lack perseverance and grit. When frustrated or challenged, they tend to give up easily. They may also be described by others as somewhat lazy. They avoid work and chores and complain more frequently than others when forced to do them. These are also the children who wail uncontrollably at their vaccinations, or when otherwise injured. Though it is normal for children to cry when hurt, most children will also respond at least at some level to efforts to provide comfort and reassurance. Children with unresolved analgesic/comfort needs, however, are inconsolable. In fact, they may flee, hit, spit, or otherwise engage in dangerous/seriously inappropriate behavior to escape pain. The threat of pain overrides all other psychological needs.

Given this need is present before birth, children are challenged to resolve it from the very beginning of their lives. And, in fact, much of childhood is naturally designed to program into children the idea that life hurts sometimes. Being born can't feel very good, but it's an immediate lesson that sometimes one must endure pain in order to encounter and experience new and wonderful things. Babies get that lesson over and over again throughout the first few years of life. When I'm hungry, I get food (which can taste *amazing*). When I fall and get a boo-boo, my mommy picks me up and gives me hugs and kisses. When I go to the doctor, I get a cool lollipop or toy. These lessons, and many more, teach children how to find balance in their analgesia/comfort needs. Still, some children, despite the early lessons, can end up with unresolved analgesia/comfort needs. Further, some of these children will present for psychotherapy. When this happens, a key mechanism of change in that psychotherapy will be to help the child reconcile these needs and move them toward a healthy balance.

Need for power: dunamis and exousia needs

All humans also need to feel at least a small amount of power. They need to feel like they have agency in their world, that they can do something themselves to meet their own needs. The Greek word *dunamis* is the root for our English words "dynamite, dynamo, and dynamic," all of which help capture the meaning of the original term, which here refers to the fact that all humans have an inherent potential, by simple virtue of being, to do all kinds of things (both good and bad). In physics terms, *dunamis* is like potential energy. *Exousia*, on the other hand, translates to "authority." It is more like a jurisdiction or dominion of influence over something else. One can have *dunamis* without *exousia*, but not the other way around (because *dunamis* is inherently present in everything – it is impossible to have "none" of it).

From a psychological perspective, humans are driven both toward exercising their inherent potential *and* toward authoritative control over others. We need to feel like we can do at least some of the things we put our energy toward and that at least someone, somewhere will listen to what we have to say and/or follow what we do. When these psychological needs are not met, humans will act in predictable ways to try to bring them back into balance. They may try to control every aspect of their life (and of the lives of others). They may develop narcissistic beliefs – that they are quasi-omnipotent or that they somehow were blessed with more *dunamis* at birth than others. Such beliefs can, at times, translate to tragic consequences, perhaps that, by blood, one race of people is inherently better than another, and that the other race needs to be eradicated. On the other end of the spectrum, unresolved power needs can lead someone toward low self-esteem or a poor sense of self-agency. They may believe they have no ability to change their life. They may become defeated and feel helpless.

A recognition of the basic human need for power drives therapists to look for such behavioral and psychological cues as those described above. They then must act, again, in a way to help resolve those power needs and move them toward a healthier central balance.

Superego needs

Defined previously, the superego acts to tell our psyche what we "should" be doing, based on interpersonal, cultural, societal, and other environmental norms/demands. Specifically, the superego is a person's own internal perception of what environmental demands mandate. Some people are driven strongly by superego demands. These people tend to always follow the "rules." In fact, they may be excessively "rules-based," unwilling to waver from expectations and unable to deviate from the "script" of whatever they are doing at the time. They may also be excessively self-sacrificing, doing things constantly for others and never catering to their own self-interests. Other people may have very weak superego drive. These people tend to follow instinct and self-interest above all else. They eschew rules and other guidelines. They may even be outright oppositional and/or antisocial.

It is widely believed that superego needs develop most strongly during toddlerhood and early childhood. When toddlers become mobile, they also become increasingly able to exercise their independence from caregivers and from authority. They can now explore their world on their own (even if doing so may be terrifying for both the toddler and the parent). There is a reason the third year of life is called the "terrible twos" and that any parent of a three-year-old can tell you about their child's "threenager" tendencies. It's because this is the stage in which children are first learning there is actually a difference between what they want to do and what they should do. Ideally, during this stage, parents scaffold children's experiences by allowing them some independence, but with safe boundaries and reasonable confines. Parents should not hover excessively, but should be vigilant to keep the environment safe enough to allow relatively free explorations. They should be available for children when the children become uneasy or anxious in their independence and need to return to the "safe base" of parents. But they should also help their children recognize that the children have agency to meet their own needs at times.

Still, some children, for any multitude of reasons, may develop imbalanced superego needs. If an imbalance does occur, again, the therapist must assume some responsibility for helping the child move toward a healthier resolution of this superego need.

Need for love

All humans need love, and all children's first loves will be their first caregiver. Love is complex to define from a scientific perspective, and that is actually okay, because all humans already possess some intuitive sense of what love is or is supposed to be anyway. In other words, love, and the capacity to feel it and experience it, are instinctual. Granted, some definitions of love can be "tainted" by extreme negative experiences. This is especially true of children with intense and/or prolonged or repeated interpersonal trauma from caregivers, who can develop an internal conflict between their instinctual sense of love compared to their lived experience of it. Still, even in those cases, the instinct to love and be loved remains. It is from this instinct that the psychological need for love derives. The need for love is present from birth but grows increasingly complex over time.

In infancy, love is experienced through normal symbiosis (see Mahler & Furer, 1968), in which, psychologically, the newborn infant is said to be unable to separate the existence of the Self from the existence of Mother (in this case, Mother is the archetypal mother, meaning whatever Object is playing the role of mother, regardless of whether this is actually a biological mother). Normal symbiosis is a theoretical construct that is impossible to prove empirically, and thus it does deserve some skepticism as to its actual validity. However, regardless of validity, the concept of normal symbiosis captures some important ideas that assist clinicians in understanding origins of the need for love and the need for Objects (see below). Importantly, normal symbiosis depicts the innate reciprocity that drives human experience throughout our existence.[4] That is, we as humans are born to be in relationship with other humans. It is our nature, and we cannot escape it without significant psychological cost.

There are common cues in childhood (and in adulthood too) that signify a possible pathology driven by insecurity in the need for love. When exploring school-related anxiety, for example, such children may express a fear that if they achieve poor grades, their parents will be angry with them. Though having a loved one be angry with you is a far leap from a literal loss of love, the worry about harming or disappointing a loved one is driven by the need to love and be loved. Of course, worry about loved ones is a normal part of the experience of love. To love is to make oneself vulnerable to caring enough about another person to spend time worrying about them. So, it is not pathological for a child simply to worry about disappointing their parents. Nonetheless, such a worry can turn pathological when it becomes excessive. So, excessive school anxiety may manifest as a child worrying constantly about grades. They stress themselves out so much about school that it becomes all-encompassing. They work hard to achieve the highest possible academic standard, all in an effort to please their parents. Sometimes, this anxiety is driven by parents who put excessive pressure on their children. Other times, children exert that pressure themselves. Still, for some, a therapist who looks hard enough may find that this school anxiety is driven by excessive loss of love anxiety. In such cases, the therapist then knows to intervene to resolve that loss of love anxiety. They are no longer acting simply to resolve school anxiety, per se; rather, they act to treat the source.

Need for Objects

Humans don't just need to love, they also need somebody (or something) to love. Imbalance in the need for an Object most often presents through Object impermanence or other types of Object insecurity. So, children can worry about loss of love, as described above, but they can also worry about loss of Objects. Separation anxiety is the classic form of Object impermanence, and this presents differently at different ages. Young children are more prone to traditional separation anxiety, where there is excessive fear and distress when literally separated from a caregiver/loved one. Older children show Object-loss anxiety through worry about something bad happening to loved ones or to themselves that may separate them from loved ones. They ask, "What if my grandmother gets sick and dies?" or, "What if Dad is in a car accident?" They may also ask, "What if I'm kidnapped and never get to see my family again?" In all these cases, the worry is driven by the fear of Object loss, without consequent loss of love fears.

Need for Objects is usually resolved through the development of Object permanence. Thus, one task for therapists is to help children establish comfort with knowing they can take loved ones with them everywhere they go, internally. There is an immense security in knowing that Objects can stay with us even when they are gone, and many spiritual traditions provide some reassurance in this area, with the knowledge that loved ones may be reunited in the spiritual world. Therapists themselves are even tasked with helping children move toward Object permanence of the therapist. In this way, children and other clients do not become dependent on the constant physical presence of the therapist to enjoy therapeutic gains. Instead, the child internalizes the therapist into their psyche, which provides therapeutic direction even when the actual therapist Object is not around.

Popularity needs

Popularity needs are almost identical to loss of love needs, but in this case the Object/source of the loss of love is not a primary attachment figure. Popularity needs are driven by the fact that humans need a variety of social contacts, not just attachment figures or Objects to love. Evolutionarily speaking, humans are "pack" animals, and for this reason, our brains are biologically and psychologically wired for functioning in groups. Furthermore, this group mentality predisposes us to both cooperation and competition, both of which are healthy for us in proper doses, but potentially toxic at improper doses. A person who is overly cooperative exercises no independence. They always follow the group, even when doing so does not serve them directly. They base too many of their decisions on whether or not the group agrees or will accept them. A person can also become excessively unconcerned with popularity needs. In such individuals, peer pressures and peer concerns rarely influence individual behavior. They often fail to consider how their actions affect others, and they ignore the collective needs of the group.

Popularity needs are heavily influenced by culture as well. The USA, for example, is a heavily individualistic culture, though there are collectivistic subcultures within the USA (e.g., Appalachian culture is notably collectivistic). Still, children who grow up in the USA hear messages throughout their life about rugged individualism and the infinite possibilities of capitalistic wealth. They are pushed to achieve and are likely to hear multiple times throughout their development that one's worth is at least partially defined by one's achievements. In other cultures, collectivistic needs take precedence, where a person's individual worth is defined not by the Self but by the value of the group and of society as a whole. In such societies, it can be said, in fact, that there "is no Self" or that the Self is an illusion (see definitions of *anatta* in Buddhist philosophy). Both of these contrasting ideals – individualism versus collectivism – create tension for children when figuring out where they, themselves, want to fall in their own value system. What matters most to them? Their own needs? Or the needs of the group? Or do both matter equally?

Competition is also driven by the group-mindedness associated with popularity needs. However, competition is often an exertion of power, and thus, competitiveness that runs rampant and unchecked can often be attributed to the need for power, as outlined above. In other words, competitiveness is a problem of power overpowering the need for popularity within a relationship. Both cooperation and competition come from our social instincts as a species, but each is a manifestation of a different psychological need.

At some point, children do begin to internalize popularity ideals into their internal psyche. Popularity needs seem to be especially heightened in adolescence, when social comparisons and peer relations become paramount in cognitive development (see Chapter 3). But popularity needs are also present much earlier, from the start of early elementary age, and persist throughout much of a person's life, to varying degrees. Unresolved popularity needs translate often to a person having too much or too little cooperation or competition. Cues of unresolved popularity needs include anxiety about social comparisons or other types of social anxieties. However, notably, social anxiety is *not always* a manifestation of popularity needs. Sometimes, social anxieties can be driven by fear of losing one's place or role in a societal hierarchy. So, a child may avoid interaction with certain peers because they see those peers as being "beneath" them – a problem of power, rather than popularity. Similarly, a child may worry about doing poorly on a test because they identify in their school as the "smart kid," and if they fail a test they will no longer be the "smart kid." By losing this "role," they are losing the identity and power associated with it, which can be deemed a crisis of that need for power. If, instead, their internal thoughts about failing the test are focused on ridicule from their friends, this would constitute a popularity crisis.

Integration needs

Integration needs are the most advanced psychological need on this list. The need for a well-integrated Self was outlined in Chapter 3, and thus I will not repeat again extensively here. To review briefly, though, a disjointed or fragmented Self can manifest in crises of identity or "set switching." Children with fragmented selves tend to present with inconsistent depictions of their own competencies and traits. When describing the Self, they fail to understand that nuances of the Self are normal and healthy, and instead they see their own idiosyncrasies as misrepresentations of the Self. They become excessively embarrassed by behaviors they feel do not reflect their nature, and they oversimplify the Self in an attempt to categorize the Self into meaningful "boxes" (e.g., they may identify as a "smart" person, and thus not allow themselves to do things a "not smart" person might do). Using an example from above, the "smart kid" that pressures themselves to achieve excellent grades on everything may do so because they believe that excellent grades are what makes them "smart." A lower-than-desired grade may then be seen as an aberration of the Self, which makes them question if they were ever such a "smart person" in the first place. Such thinking can drive people toward a disintegration crisis (albeit a relatively mild one), where they must figure out how to reconcile this aberrant behavior with their internal identity.

Humans may engage in a variety of defense mechanisms to protect themselves and/or resolve a disintegration crisis. Freud and other psychoanalytic therapists have written extensively about defense mechanisms, a full exploration of which is beyond the scope of this book. However, a few examples include denial, repression, regression, and reaction formation. In denial, the person may simply deny any aberration of the Self ever happened. "I didn't fail that test – they must have graded it wrong or something!" or, "The machine that grades those must have been broken." Out of their denial, they may demand a "recount" or "regrade," or they may simply just move on, living in denial without challenging the outcome. In repression, the person not only denies the facts, but seems to even "forget" that they ever happened. In their mind, the failed test never happened, because they are a "smart person" and "smart people don't fail tests." When asked, they may say things such as, "I've never failed anything," and they'll actually believe it, because their mind has repressed all failures.

In regression, a person reverses maturity a bit to resolve a psychological crisis. To cope with failing the test, they may throw a tantrum (a regression to the *anal* [5] stage, representing a loss of control) or may soothe themselves through drinking alcohol (a regression to *oral* needs, representing dependence). Such regressions resort to immature coping skills to escape a crisis, rather than facing it. Lastly, in reaction formation, a person focuses excessive mental energy toward the *opposite* internal reaction. So, if failing the test made them feel stupid, they may respond with a reaction formation to engage in an excessive number of "smart" things. They study for hours on end, post to social media some intellectual manifesto barely understood by most of their peers, or proclaim loudly to their brother, "I'm still smarter than *you*!"

Regardless of what defenses are used, most are aimed at preserving the integrity of the Self, even if doing so comes at a cost. Thus, one mechanism of change in psychotherapy is focused on helping people unify the Self without having to resort to (psychologically) costly defenses. Instead, the therapist helps the client replace defenses with healthy coping skills designed to accept reality and accommodate a new Self that can respond properly to the reality around it.

Other core psychoanalytic ideas influencing how change occurs in psychotherapy

Analytic theory also gives us a number of developmental stages that are frequently used to guide therapists in executing the mechanism of re-experiencing and working through. In describing stages, I will use some of the original Freudian terms so that readers may appreciate their history, but I find a more modernized version of the stages to be more acceptable to analytically untrained audiences, and so I will also translate to the modern language.

The oral stage of development is the most primitive. It was termed "oral" because it occurs during infancy, when babies experience much of the world (and much comfort) through their mouths – through breastfeeding, suckling, or just general mouthing. In modern terms, the oral stage represents dependence. During infancy, babies are completely dependent on others to provide for their needs. Sure, they can cry to get someone's attention, but without a caregiver to give them what they need, they will die. Thus, the oral stage reflects a person's relative level of dependence on others. One can be overly dependent or overly independent. An *oral fixation*, in classic usage, simply refers to a person who remains overly dependent past the stage in which oral dependence is supposed to present – that is, past infancy. In the example above, where *oral regression* was referenced in the context of alcohol abuse during times of stress, the person is seeking to meet their needs through alcohol/drug use. In other words, they are dependent upon alcohol to reduce distress, unable to cope on their own. As with all dynamic needs, the key to healthy functioning is balance, and so the goal of maturity is for a person to be able to depend on others at times but also be capable of independence when necessary or useful.

The anal stage of development comes next. The term "anal" is given because the stage occurs during toddlerhood, during which potty training occurs. Anal needs, then, refer to a person's ability to exert control, to withhold satisfaction of their needs until the proper place and time. To potty train properly, a child learns to hold back their bowel and bladder movements until they are on the potty, putting both where they belong. A person can fault on both ends of the anal control spectrum, either holding things in so much that they become constipated (figuratively) or releasing things with so little control that they are (again, figuratively) pooping all over the place. If we follow the metaphor fully, a person who is *anal retentive*, then, is a person who feels such a strong need for control that they hold in all their needs until they become constipated. They are unable to relax, and, as such, get "backed up" with stress until they are eventually overwhelmed. For this reason, *anal retentive* people tend to experience high amounts of stress and frequently feel as if they are on the verge of exploding. On the other end of the spectrum, a person can also be *anal expletive*, in which case they are just letting themselves go anywhere and everywhere, regardless of the consequences or effects on other people. Such people often lack emotional control and tend to release their feelings without any filter. This can be particularly problematic if that uncontrolled feeling is anger, because uncontrolled release of anger often results in antisocial behaviors toward others (fighting, shouting, cursing, etc.).

The phallic stage comes next in development, occurring in preschool and early elementary age. This stage relates originally to gender identity and sexuality. It derives its name from the fact that this is the stage in which children first develop a sense of differences between males and females, and from the fact that Freud (I believe) wanted to keep a consistent theme of bodily themes in his psychosexual stages (otherwise he could have termed it the "identity" stage). Children during the phallic stage, now able to notice differences between males and females, also start to identify personal characteristics they have themselves that also make them male or female. If we ignore, though, what is often judged by others as being an over-focus on sexuality in Freud's original theories, we can view a modern version of this stage as being primarily about the first stages of identity. During the phallic stage, children develop a primitive, emerging sense of identity. As described in Chapter 3, early childhood identities are usually simple, concrete, and rely heavily on (observable) physical characteristics, and then they become more complex over time.

Problems can emerge in the phallic stage when a person over-identifies with a limited aspect of their overall identity. For example, a young child may have aspects of the Self that are like Dad and some that are like Mom. However, during their phallic stage, they may over-identify with Dad and seek to be more like him, perhaps even forgoing some of their natural inclinations. Naturally, the child may not be terribly driven toward sports. They may prefer music, but, if Dad likes sports, they may try to build sports into their own identity in order to be more like Dad. Over time, they could even make themselves miserable by continuing in sports that they hate out of an effort to fit the identity they feel they should fit to be like Dad, even if in reality Dad does not care whether or not the child likes sports. In the FELT framework, phallic problems most often fall under the rubric of "integration needs," but may also carry some flavor of "loss of love" or "loss of Object" needs.

The next psychosexual stage was the latency stage, called such because, well, not much was happening sexually during that time, and so it was a latency between phallic and the later genital stage (see below). In reality, a lot does happen psychologically during the latency phase, which was reviewed in Chapter 3. It is during latency that identities get challenged and grow increasingly complex. The reader is referred to Chapter 3 to review more of the psychological processes that occur in middle to late childhood.

The final psychosexual stage is called the genital stage, which starts at puberty and continues through adulthood. During the genital stage, (most) humans can now reproduce, and so analysts focus this stage on a person's relative activity in creating, sustaining, and enhancing life (for the Self and for

Others). This is the "final destination" of psychological maturity, in which the core goals of development have been attained and now the person can focus on building their life and on psychological fulfillment.

Many of these Freudian psychosexual stages overlap with Erik Erikson's theories of psychosocial development, published in the late 1950s and early 1960s. Erikson's psychosocial "stages" also focused on "crises" of development that needed resolution in order to promote optimal psychological functioning. So, in place of Freud's *oral* needs, Erikson called the first psychosocial crisis one of "trust versus mistrust," where children find how much they can rely on others to provide for their needs. Freud's *anal* stage is most analogous to "autonomy versus shame" in Erikson's model. In autonomy versus shame, though, there is less focus on the ability for control than there is on the transition from dependence to independence. So, children have to answer the questions, "Can I do things on my own, and, when I do, can I do them right? Do others have confidence in my ability to meet my own needs?" The next childhood Eriksonian stage is initiative versus guilt. This stage focuses on assertiveness. Once a child has moved through autonomy versus shame, building a basic trust in self-competence (or not), they must now identify if they can use that competence to achieve meaningful objectives without overstepping the basic autonomy and rights of others. Children can succeed or fail on multiple levels here – on achieving the actual objective and/or on respecting others while doing so. Failures on either can lead to guilt.

The next Eriksonian stage is industry versus inferiority, which occurs in elementary school-aged children, and which we analyzed extensively previously in this chapter. This is the stage in which children build their capacity for specific competencies and comparison to others, which leads them in turn to finding what they're good at (industry) and what they're not good at (inferiority). As noted earlier, the healthy norm for children here is for them to lean toward generally positive views of the Self. If inferiority predominates, this increases risk for various forms of psychopathology.

The final Eriksonian stage relevant in FELT is identity versus role confusion, which typifies adolescence and so typically does not emerge in children to whom FELT is commonly applied. But identity and role confusion *can* develop before adolescence in some cases, and so I will review it briefly here. During this stage, children build and solidify their basic identity. They are exploring different parts of their identity and the roles they want to fill in their lives. For this reason, adolescents commonly "experiment" with different roles and peer groups, trying to find what fits them best. Most youth, by late adolescence (17–18), build a more solid sense of Self and can elaborate basically who they are and who they expect to be long term. This stage can sometimes be prolonged a bit during college or other early vocational explorations, as emerging and young adults grapple with larger societal roles within the adult world. At the early stages (around ages 11–13), children are still branching out and typically unable to express a unified, integrated identity. Thus, this step maps most closely to "integration needs" referenced previously. In FELT, it is not expected that children will resolve this stage, but they may routinely be encouraged to explore multiple aspects of the Self while being introduced to the concept that containing multiple "Me's" is normal.

Insight, re-experiencing, and working through: summary

In summary, the mechanisms involved in helping clients gain insight, re-experience, and work through developmental/psychological needs are complex, yet key to a thorough understanding of how meaningful change occurs in psychotherapy. A skilled FELT therapist should have a firm grasp of these psychodynamic needs, how to identify them, and how to help children then move toward balance in each need. In FELT, identifying patterns in psychodynamic development is one of the most essential components used to inform client-specific goals in targeted sessions during the latter half of an intervention. So, it is fundamental for a therapist practicing FELT to consider the universal psychological needs of humans and to develop concrete plans for addressing those needs during session.

Problem-solving techniques and coping strategies

The next mechanism of therapeutic change is a practical, solution-focused one. A substantial amount of change in psychotherapy occurs through the direct learning and practice of coping strategies and problem-solving skills. Therapists enact change by teaching healthy coping techniques to clients and helping them execute the techniques reliably and with fidelity. The mechanisms and interventions used are often derived from empirically supported practices and cognitive-behavioral traditions. Because skills-based approaches are the most concrete of all the mechanisms of change, they are the easiest to research. It is extremely difficult, for example, to measure empirically whether a true catharsis or corrective emotional experience occurred, and psychodynamic theories are profoundly complex and multilayered, making them nearly impossible to track in a research study. Coping skills and problem-solving, though, can be tracked much more easily. They can also be taught to therapists quite easily, which, again, helps empiricism because it allows for less variability among therapists in a treatment study *and* requires less time to train them in a specific intervention.

Recent research advancements have allowed for a somewhat transdiagnostic depiction of specific coping strategies that seem to be effective with most child patients, regardless of presenting problem/diagnosis. One universally effective coping strategy is the concept that changing thoughts tremendously increases chances of changing emotions. Cognitive therapy is present in every empirically supported, effective approach to modern psychotherapy, and for good reason – it just works. The techniques through which thought-changing is accomplished differ among various approaches, with many using specific written exercises and giving children "homework" to practice those exercises outside of session, whereas others (including FELT) approach thought-changing mainly through modeling, support, and teaching other mental relaxation strategies (such as storytelling or meditation) to address mental activity. Even prayer can be a form of effective cognitive therapy for many, especially for those who use prayer as a means to express and experience hope and optimism about future outcomes.

Another rather universal coping strategy includes goal-directed (rather than mood-directed) behaviors. Helping clients focus their behaviors to be more consistent with healthy, long-term goals, rather than being controlled by mood, is another key to promoting optimal functioning. Therapists often start by first identifying specific, healthy, long-term goals, and then they help clients execute working toward those goals. In treating anxiety, for example, therapists teach clients to practice daily relaxation/stress-relieving behaviors, which will vary by client, depending on their interests. If a client wants to be social, but has social anxiety, the therapist helps them identify ways they can challenge themselves to pursue social interests, without letting anxiety stop them, and while teaching other strategies to keep social anxiety manageable during those social pursuits. Similar examples can be offered for other psychiatric conditions too. Still, the act of creating an intent to change, and then pursuing that intent through behavioral efforts is another universal coping skill.

Increasing social support is yet another universal coping skill. Clients are known to do better and experience longer-lasting gains when they have partners to help them in their journey to improve. In child psychotherapy, there are often multiple possible social supports present, including parents, teachers, coaches, siblings, friends, and more. Children are encouraged to use those supports routinely to help maximize maintenance of gains in therapy.

Object-relations, internal representations, and interpersonal development

This mechanism of change focuses on the attributes of the therapeutic relationship itself that help manifest therapeutic growth. There is much research that supports the idea that without some baseline necessary conditions within a therapeutic relationship, a therapist cannot be effective. I dedicate an entire chapter in this book (Chapter 5) to exploring the core principles of effective therapy, which includes extensive discussion on the importance of a therapeutic relationship and other interpersonal factors in psychotherapy, and so I divert the reader to Chapter 5 for a more extensive review of these relationship-based factors of change. For now, it is sufficient simply to know that a major portion of change that occurs in therapy is achieved directly through interpersonal processes that occur between the client and therapist within various therapeutic exchanges.

Overlapping mechanisms in integrative therapy

The five broad mechanisms typically function simultaneously throughout a therapeutic intervention. Over the course of therapy, therapists will help their clients express emotions, serve as a container for those emotions, generate new insights, work through unresolved psychological conflicts, teach problem-solving techniques and coping skills, and relate to the client in ways designed to facilitate therapeutic growth. Regardless of their identified orientation or school of training, these mechanisms of change occur in any therapeutic exchange. The simultaneity of these processes makes them impossible to parse empirically. In other words, our science is unable to quantify any incremental differences, if any, each mechanism makes in generating real change for clients. The questions of how much coping skills matter, compared to, say, insights and working through will probably never be answered satisfactorily, because the very act of teaching coping skills also involves working through conflict, and vice versa. There is an argument, then, that perhaps the various mechanisms listed in this chapter are all necessary components of a whole, each unable to function without the others. Alternatively, the differences may simply be in semantics – that is, they are different ways of describing the same thing.

However, therapists are most effective when they do consciously identify the mechanisms of change they target in therapy (Wampold, 2001). For this reason, therapists who implement FELT should achieve at least a baseline competence in all the above mechanisms. In particular, it is essential for FELT therapists to be able to use planned interventions to push change in individual clients based on an individualized case conceptualization. Given a set of predictors that drives the psychopathology of any given client, therapists must be able to intervene at each predictor/risk factor, in order to maximize the effect of psychotherapy. The FELT case conceptualization model and processes for identifying specific needs within clients are outlined in Chapter 6.

Notes

1 Russ technically described six mechanisms of change, the five described herein plus a sixth factor she called "nonspecific variables" and which she listed as including "expectation of change, hope, awareness of parental concern, and no longer feeling so alone" (2004, p. 41). In FELT, most of these characteristics are captured under the Object-relations framework described in Chapter 3, where a goal for change is to help the client establish healthy Self- and Object representations.
2 From Greek, *dunamis* is most often translated as "power, potential, or ability," whereas *exousia* is most often translated as "authority." Humans have a need to feel at least some level of both.
3 Though this is certainly an empirical question – one could measure it – I am not aware of any studies that have actually done so. Thus, these "guesses" are based on anecdotal clinical experience.
4 This concept of how relationships shape brain development and human personality is outlined extensively in the seminal work by Dr. Dan Siegel, *The Developing Mind* (1999).
5 These terms – the anal and oral stages – are defined further in the next section.

REFERENCES

Craig, K. D., Whitfield, M. F., Grunau, R. V. E., Linton, J., & Hadjistavropoulos, H. D. (1993). Pain in the preterm neonate: behavioural and physiological indices. *Pain*, 52(3), 287–299.

Mahler, M. S., & Furer, M. (1968). *On Human Symbiosis and the Vicissitudes of Individuation: I. Infantile Psychosis*. Madison, CT: International Universities Press.

Russ, S. W. (2004). *Play in Child Development and Psychotherapy: Toward Empirically Supported Practice*. Mahwah, NJ: Erlbaum.

Slater, R., Cantarella, A., Gallella, S., Worley, A., Boyd, S., Meek, J., & Fitzgerald, M. (2006). Cortical pain responses in human infants. *Journal of Neuroscience*, 26 (14), 3662–3666.

Wampold, B. (2001). *The Great Psychotherapy Debate: Models, Methods, and Findings*. Mahwah, NJ: Erlbaum.

Chapter 5

Core principles of effective therapy
The ACER characteristics

An analysis of the mechanisms of change discussed in Chapter 4 reveals a list of common techniques used to facilitate change through each mechanism (see Russ, 2004). Under expression/catharsis, therapists use techniques such as giving clients permission and space to express themselves safely. They also help clients label their emotions and accept those emotions as being valid and real. Therapists may also communicate understanding, empathy, and strength to help bring about a corrective emotional experience. Analytic mechanisms, by definition, push therapists to assist clients with making interpretations of their lived experiences, both conscious and unconscious. They may use modeling, active teaching, role play, rehearsing, and homework as means to build reliable use of coping skills. Lastly, to strengthen interpersonal processes, therapists may use empathy, caring, and genuineness.

In FELT, these core techniques are summarized under the ACER model: *attunement, concern, expertise*, and *responsivity*. We will explore each of these individually below. In order to maximize the execution of effective therapy, therapists should consistently strive to implement the ACER characteristics in every interaction with clients and their parents.

Attunement

Attunement refers to efforts by the therapist to communicate empathy, caring, and connection with the internal state of the child client. A frequent metaphor used in describing attunement refers to attunement being like "tuning in" to the radio frequency of the patient. An attuned therapist, then, is "dialed in with," "on the same page as," or "in harmony with" their patient. I prefer, however, a different definition. I think of attunement as being "at-one-ment," because "at-one-ment" communicates that the therapist is not only listening or working in harmony with the patient, but also using a relational connection to merge, psychologically, in some ways with the patient. Through this psychological merging, therapists are not only better connected to their clients, better able to understand their plight and follow their direction, but they are also able to effect change directly by imparting some of their own

DOI: 10.4324/9781032693187-6

psychological stability onto the client. In other words, by being "at one" with the client, the therapist themself is also inviting the client to join in being "at one" with them. When the client is so joined, the therapist can then project some healthier internal ideals into the client, such that when the connection is severed, that patient still carries some of those internal projections with them (a process called projective identification). So, attunement involves far more than listening with empathy and care, it involves intimate connection between the therapist and the patient.

Accurate attunement facilitates all other aspects of the therapeutic process. It is only after attunement that a therapist can facilitate labeling of emotions, especially in children, whose own immature emotional intelligence and weaker verbal skills limit their ability to communicate their own emotions in traditional ways. Through attunement, a therapist can shape a child's understanding of their own emotions. Furthermore, attunement requires attentiveness to the child client. Renowned teacher and religious scholar Simone Weil wrote extensively about attention being a practice of open-mindedness and intrigue. Weil believed that we (humans) do not gain insights by going in search of them, but rather by waiting for them. As described by her biographer Zaretsky (2021), Weil further writes that attention requires letting go of (attention to) the self, and "allowing the other to grab [our] full attention." In this manner, attention is a way to show others a deep care and concern for them. By attending to a child client, a therapist is communicating, "You matter!" and that, "I am here for whatever you need right now!" Both are powerful messages for growth.

Similarly, an attuned therapist communicates positive regard for the patient. Carl Rogers wrote extensively about the power of unconditional positive regard in helping patients (Rogers, 1956). A therapist who does not hold their patient in positive regard may unconsciously bias themselves toward negative attributions about the patient and/or may tend to wane in attentiveness toward the patient, exhausted by their own disregard. For this reason, a therapist's unconditional positive regard for their patients drives them toward attunement, and accurate attunement can only happen if the therapist experiences a genuine care for the patient. Now, that care does not need to be personal. In fact, a therapist who maintains boundaries between professional and personal is usually able to perform better and maintain proper therapeutic ethics. So, professional care is enough.

Attunement also boosts accuracy of insights and interpretations of a child's play. Attunement is a reciprocal, flexible process. In other words, an attuned therapist interprets a child's behaviors and communications and helps children and their parents make sense of their internal experiences, but through attunement, the therapist also leaves room for themselves to be wrong about initial impressions and adapts their findings and approach according to ongoing feedback from children and their families.

Concern

A professional therapeutic relationship is not a friendship. It was instituted in order to help a patient with a specific problem. Thus, from the onset of the professional relationship, it is a relationship formed out of concern. The therapist is concerned about the patient's ultimate welfare and assumes a responsibility to facilitate therapeutic change. When it comes to Play Therapy, in particular, children often blur the line between "play" and "therapy." Many children call their play therapist a "play buddy," and they come to see therapy as a time to have fun with an adult who enjoys playing with them. In such cases, it is often up to the therapist, then, to maintain sufficient concern to help keep everyone focused on the purpose of sessions, which is to address the presenting problem (and any underlying risk factors). It is out of concern, then, that therapists establish a therapeutic contract with children and their parents. They then follow that contract throughout treatment, adapting it as necessary as new treatment needs arise or old ones resolve.

Importantly, though, the concerned therapist need not be serene or unwilling to waver momentarily from the task at hand. Children will engage in some level of frivolity in therapy, and it's okay for therapists to let their child clients enjoy some unfocused silliness at times. Although a concerned therapist should eventually try to "rein things in" and get to work, children can also be allowed momentary deviations from the therapy contract, especially if other indicators signify a potential need for a "break" from an emotionally intense session.

Therapists communicate concern through curiosity. The curious therapist seeks to understand the child. They inquire into multiple domains of the child's life, wanting to know them as a whole person and never being satisfied with a cursory picture of just the child and the reason they came to therapy. Through curiosity, an effective therapist builds a more informed case conceptualization to guide treatment, and treats children as being more than just their diagnosis.

A therapist is also cautious. Rather than make interpretations, they make interpretive *guesses*, allowing the client and therapist to correct inaccurate interpretations when they do inevitably "miss the mark." They proceed with respect for the patient's and parents' readiness to engage in different tiers of therapeutic intensity. When a child becomes overwhelmed with overly intense therapy, the therapist backs off a bit and reassesses how to prepare the child for the next steps. This cautiousness is thus balanced with concern, therapist and patient engaged in a "dance" toward meeting therapeutic goals without pushing one before they are ready.

Expertise

A child therapist should also be an expert in clinical psychology and counseling theory and in child/human development. Much of this expertise is achieved through initial academic preparation for licensure (i.e., an advanced degree) and through continuing education relevant to their field of practice. A substantial portion of this book is dedicated to ensuring therapists have the requisite academic background and expertise to execute effective therapy, but background coursework in counseling theory, empirical practice, and child development are usually additional prerequisites to being able to fully digest the clinical applications of FELT. Still, the point of this domain is that a skilled therapist requires extensive, specialized training.

Expertise is required not only for understanding how variations in child development interact with the application of therapeutic principles; a therapist should also be well-versed in psychopathology (Chapter 6) and in etiological models of various childhood psychiatric complaints. Given etiological models do vary across psychiatric conditions, and given FELT has been studied exclusively in relation to anxiety so far, FELT should not be seen at this time as being broadly applicable in its current form to every child who presents for psychotherapy. Though the FELT model can be adapted to fit multiple etiological paradigms, the conceptualization model outlined in this book is specific to anxiety. Still, expert therapists can adapt FELT techniques to fit individual client needs. Doing so holds consistent with the goal to manualize a "contextual" approach to practice.

Responsivity

It is not enough to be attuned, concerned, and an expert, a therapist must also actively respond to a client's needs and their own goals/direction. A responsive therapist modifies their own directiveness or non-directiveness based on the expressed needs of the child (see Benedict, 2003). Interventions are chosen specifically "in attuned responsiveness to the child's play and patterns of interactions with the therapist" (Benedict, 2003, p. 289). The story stem format of FELT is designed to facilitate a healthy balance in directiveness versus non-directiveness. So, the therapist chooses and designs story stems in real time based on a child's given needs each session, and then the therapist must respond appropriately to themes that arise in the child's continuation of the story. In this manner, therapists are able to respond both to a child's overall clinical needs *and* to the specific content they bring into session each week. Importantly, responsivity requires accurate attunement. It also occurs directly out of concern, and it requires expertise. Thus, responsivity is seen as a culminating action that feeds directly from the other ACE characteristics, a necessary, inevitable reaction that follows logically from being an attuned, concerned expert.

In FELT, therapists most commonly respond directly through and within the play-based realm. Interventions are administered through play and play-based commentary. Occasionally, though, a child may demonstrate a need and/or readiness for alternative forms of intervention, including more direct talk therapy. Just because FELT is designed as a play therapy does not mean that a therapist cannot deviate from the *format* of therapy in attuned responsivity to a client's needs. In other words, the ACER characteristics and the overarching goals of therapeutic change are more important than sticking to the play and conducting play analysis. At the same time, it would also be imprudent for a responsive therapist to never engage in play with a young child, because evading play in most young children would be inconsistent with developmental needs. Responsive therapists, then, must balance their responses to multiple "directions" in a therapeutic session, wagering their response to overall clinical needs against immediate, live-in-session content against a child's developmental capacities and preferences, and against the goals of parents (which at times may not be fully consistent with actual clinical needs).

A therapist is never perfect in balancing all these responses, either. There will be times when a planned intervention proves beyond the capacity of a child's state of mind that day in session, or when logistical barriers result in improper dosing of therapy (e.g., every two weeks, instead of every one week). In such cases, a child's long-term clinical needs may take a "back seat" to immediate barriers, and a therapist may choose to address the barriers first. However, there are times that this choice may be an erroneous choice, where responding to barriers becomes a repeated focus of clinical work over months, after which it then becomes more difficult to return to the clinical need at hand. Therefore, responsive therapists must always seek opportunities to maneuver a long-term clinical need into otherwise "off-topic" interactions within therapy. If, for example, a child has had a "rough day" before their session – they have been hyper and somewhat "off the walls" all day, which continues to some degree even in your session – a therapist may use playful commentary to observe how sometimes people just feel like they are "all over the place," and may then demonstrate coping skills that help to recenter in times of behavioral disorganization. Such a demonstration would presumably connect to longer-term clinical skills of emotional and behavioral regulation. In this way, the therapist has not "abandoned" the clinical need, even if they did have to change the way they intended to execute that plan that day. Similarly, if a child's parents have barriers to attending regular appointments, therapists may work with resources in which the child does have regular interactions (e.g., school, after-school programs, etc.) to teach therapeutic skill-building inside those resources, which can help facilitate inter-session practice.

Summary

The ACER characteristics represent a framework of "common factors" (see Wampold, 2001) that guides therapists to self-monitor what they do in session that translates to clinical efficacy. ACER practices are a combination of a therapeutic philosophy and concrete behaviors. They also form a core of fidelity monitoring in FELT research. When training others in FELT, supervisors place a high value on teaching new and experienced therapists how to self-monitor for and enact the ACER characteristics in every clinical interaction. Supervisors also directly rate therapists on their implementation of these factors in fidelity checklists (see the FELT treatment fidelity checklist in Chapter 2). FELT presupposes that a therapist cannot be effective without employing the ACER characteristics at a minimum. So, for therapists considering using FELT in their own practice, it is strongly advised that they obtain supervisors or colleagues who can help monitor to maximize the execution of "common factors" and ACER characteristics through every session.

REFERENCES

Benedict, H. E. (2003). Object-relations/thematic play therapy. In C. E. Schaefer (Ed.), *Foundations of Play Therapy* (pp. 281–305). Hoboken, NJ: Wiley.

Rogers, C. (1956). *Client-Centered Therapy* (3rd ed.). Boston, MA: Houghton Mifflin.

Russ, S. W. (2004). *Play in Child Development and Psychotherapy: Toward Empirically Supported Practice*. Mahwah, NJ: Erlbaum.

Wampold, B. (2001). *The Great Psychotherapy Debate: Models, Methods, and Findings*. Mahwah, NJ: Erlbaum.

Zaretsky, R. (2021). *The Subversive Simone Weil: A Life in Five Ideas*. Chicago, IL: University of Chicago Press.

Chapter 6

FELT etiological model of anxiety

As discussed elsewhere, FELT's evidence base thus far is rooted in the treatment of children with anxiety disorders. FELT has only been researched in treating anxiety, and the etiological model presented in this chapter was designed specifically for therapist use in the treatment of anxiety. It is presented here for readers to follow the core tenets of the framework in implementing FELT with anxious children. However, it is my sincere hope that similar FELT principles can be applied across other diagnoses and presenting problems, adapting etiological models as needed. In other words, though FELT's research so far has been limited to children with clinically significant anxiety, I firmly believe the principles can apply to other presenting problems, particularly those with significant overlap with anxiety, including depression, trauma, and other stress-related disorders. Thus, in this chapter, I first review the FELT etiological model of anxiety.

The FELT anxiety model

The FELT model is a three-tier model (see Figure 6.1). The first tier is labeled *propagating factors*, which includes psychodynamic, genetic, and environmental/cultural/learned factors. Propagating factors are believed to be those features which predispose or create increased risk for a person to respond anxiously to perceived stressors. These propagating factors, when present, lead to the second tier, which is labeled *manifest factors*. Manifest factors represent the way that anxiety shows itself in any individual person and include both neurophysiological and cognitive processes. The construct of negative affect, traditionally described in other models as a trait (Costa & McCrae, 1987; Watson & Clark, 1984; Gray, 1987), is also included under manifest factors. The third tier is labeled *temporal factors*. Temporal factors refer to the effects of timing on how propagating and manifest factors function along a developmental spectrum. With children, there are certain features of anxiety which are normative at different developmental periods; thus, manifest anxiety is judged differently

DOI: 10.4324/9781032693187-7

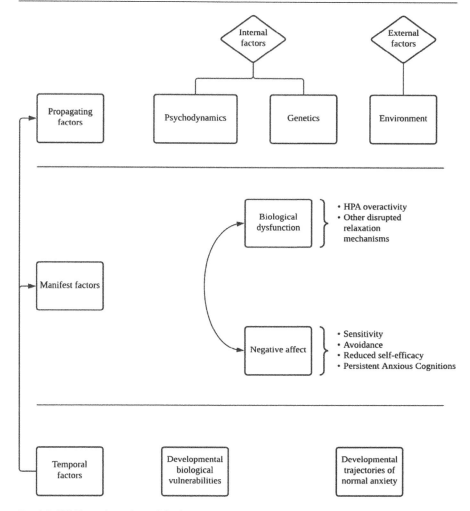

Fig. 6.1 FELT etiological model of anxiety
HPA = hypothalamic-pituitary-adrenal axis.

depending on timing of manifestation. Likewise, there are different developmental periods where exposure to certain propagating factors may have differential effects on how symptoms progress to manifest factors. Therefore, temporal factors may also affect the overall level of risk associated with any propagating factor. Each of these three tiers, along with relevant research support, as well as how each can be assessed clinically, is described more fully below.

Propagating factors

Genetic factors

The first type of propagating factors is genetic. Within the current model "genetic factors" refer to biological risks for anxiety that a child is endowed with by the end of early- to early-middle childhood (ages 5–7 years), a pinnacle time when many of the brain's major functions (excluding executive functioning) have reached biological maturity (Giedd et al., 1996; Carmichael, 1990; Pfefferbaum et al., 1994). While perhaps unusual to define genetic factors in this way, I have done so here in order to capture the complexities of the effects of gene by environment (GxE) interactions on neurobiological functioning. Scientists are now well aware that gene expression is a complex procedure that can be altered both prenatally and postnatally by environmental influences, including, but not limited to, sex, drugs/chemicals, temperature, viruses, and early rearing (Guzowski et al., 2001; Hamadeh et al., 2002; Issa, 2000; Meaney, 2010; Parsch & Ellegren, 2013; Reik & Walter, 2001; Silverman, 2004; Sturtevant, 1913; Szyf, 2009). Thus, the influence of genetics cannot be adequately or accurately understood without also appreciating the influence of environment on gene expression. Simply put, some genetic expression can be turned "on" or "off" by environmental demands, and it is during childhood that the majority of neurobiological, genetic "programming" occurs. By the end of early childhood, basic biological rhythms and emotional expression are well-established (see Siegel, 2020), and though these neural processes can be altered after early childhood, they are far more vulnerable during early development. Hence, the 0–7 age range is perhaps the most critical period to manage genetic vulnerability to anxious functioning.

For psychotherapists, the primary point of intervention at the genetic level is to implement environmental strategies that can "turn off" genetic predispositions to anxiety and "turn on" healthier alternatives. Thus, in the current model, we highlight several environmental "amplifiers" and "suppressors" that have been associated in the literature with augmenting or diminishing general anxious functioning. Amplifiers are those environmental factors which seem to amplify biological manifestations of anxiety-predisposing genetic code, while suppressors do the opposite. The primary task, then, for the genetically conscious psychotherapist is to implement interventions which work to reduce ("turn off") environmental amplifiers and enhance ("turn on") environmental suppressors. The majority of such work is completed within the remaining factors in the model, in which various amplifiers and suppressors are defined under each category. In the FELT model, I name them amplifiers and suppressors (rather than risk and protective factors) to highlight the interactive effects of these factors on basic biological/genetic functioning. Naming them in this manner more intently alerts clinicians to practice in a more integrative manner, instead of focusing too heavily on any single tier of the model (i.e., genetics/biology).

Psychodynamic factors

Psychodynamic theory posits that anxious symptomatology derives from psychic conflict that goes unresolved at various critical developmental periods (Gabbard, 2014). The logical goal, then, for clinicians who practice psychodynamic therapy within this particular point of view is to help clients resolve the conflict, which should then translate to resolution of symptoms. In line with this perspective, existing psychoanalytic and psychodynamic treatments for childhood anxiety focus on identifying and modifying a central conflict theme (Göttken et al., 2014) or using transference interpretations to increase understanding of anxiety (Milrod et al., 2013). The FELT model deviates slightly from this "classical" stance. While FELT does work under the assumption that all humans have basic psychic needs that drive behavior (see Chapter 4), and while FELT posits that people who follow extremes of psychic needs tend to more frequently exhibit psychiatric symptoms, in FELT these factors are only a part of our larger integrative model. Consequently, FELT therapists do not practice with the single underlying goal of identifying the conflict and resolving it, thereby resolving symptoms. I do, on the other hand, believe that a thorough treatment of anxiety should consider intrapsychic features which may contribute to the anxiety, and clinicians should then structure treatment in such a way as to target those underlying intrapsychic conflicts, which should then, if fully resolved, theoretically translate to decreased lifetime risk of later relapse.

The psychodynamic risk factors (intrapsychic conflicts) in the FELT model fall under six categories, and these were described in detail in Chapter 4. These are analogous to the basic human needs reviewed under the "Insight, re-experiencing, and working through" mechanism of change. For simplicity, I list these again below.

1   A need to be free from pain/comfortable (analgesia/comfort needs)
2   A need to feel at least some level of power (*dunamis* and *exousia* needs)
3   A need to meet one's own expectations for the Self (superego needs)
4   A need to be loved by others, particularly a primary attachment figure (need for love)
5   A need for something to love (need for Objects)
6   A need to be well-liked and well-received by Others who are not attachment figures (popularity needs)
7   A need for a unified, true Self (integration needs)

The analogous anxieties that are generated from irresolution of these needs are 1) castration anxiety (which includes a fear of pain and a fear of powerlessness), 2) superego anxiety, 3) loss of love anxiety, 4) loss of Object anxiety, 5) persecutory anxiety, and 6) disintegration anxiety (see also Gabbard, 2014).

Castration anxiety derives from a person's need to be free from pain and/or a person's need to feel powerful. All people have these needs; those with castration anxiety tend to focus excessive energy on fulfilling (or worrying about fulfilling) these needs. Clinically, then, castration anxiety may manifest as persistent thoughts about getting hurt or about losing power (usually within the realm of a social hierarchy). Superego anxiety stems from a person's need to meet their own Self-expectations. The anxiety then results from excessive fear or worry about failing to meet the standards of the superego. Clinically, such anxiety can present as overly negative Self-appraisals – "I'll never be able to get what I want out of life"; "I have to ace the test, or I'll hate myself."

Loss of love anxiety develops from a need to be loved by Others, particularly by a primary attachment figure. Similarly, anxiety about a loss of Object grows out of a need to have an attachment figure. While similar, loss of love and loss of Object anxieties are independent; one can worry about losing a parent's love, without simultaneously losing the parent, while one can also fear losing a parent, without simultaneously losing their love. Anxiety about loss of love often (but not always) manifests similarly to superego anxiety, but the source of the anxiety is a loved one's appraisals, rather than one's own. Therefore, underlying Self-statements may read, "I'll never ace this test, and my parents will hate me if I don't." Anxiety about loss of Object often shows up in children as separation anxiety or as fear of harm coming to loved ones – "I'm afraid I'll be kidnapped and never see my mom again"; "When Dad got sick, I thought he would die." Loss-of-Object fears are not always about *losing* the Object, per se. It can also drive fears about any harm to the Object. Kids who worry about their father getting sick, for example, need not necessarily worry that the illness will lead to his death; worries about the illness alone, and about Dad being sick, also constitute loss-of-Object fears.

Persecutory anxiety originates from a person's need to be well-liked and well-received by Others. Humans have an extremely social nature as a species, and much of our natural biology is socially dependent (Siegel, 2020). As a result, all people will, at some point in their lives, and at varying levels, pay attention to Others. Those with persecutory anxiety, however, will tend to over-focus on worry about Others' (non-loved-ones') appraisals of them. Using our same test example above, a person with persecutory anxiety may say, "If I don't ace this test, my classmates will think I'm stupid." At the farthest extreme, persecutory anxiety transitions to paranoia.

The final psychodynamic need is that of a unified, true Self. Disintegration anxiety, then, classifies fears or worries about losing one's sense of Self or losing who one really is. In classical psychodynamic theory, this type of anxiety is used to describe schizophreniform delusions and/or dissociative identity problems (Gabbard, 2014). However, there are also normative examples of disintegration anxiety. In my own work, I have seen disintegration fears frequently in the children of divorced parents, where a child may develop a need to manage different rules in different environments. It is also frequently seen in normal stages of adolescent Self-development, where teens must negotiate differences between how they represent themselves with peers at school versus with their parents at home (see Harter, 2012). Many can recognize that this is normal and not a clinical concern. However, sometimes, this negotiation process can transition to disintegration anxiety – "I *hate* that I feel fake," or, "I think a lot about Mom and Dad getting back together *so I can stop splitting myself between them.*"

In treatment, therapists may focus on psychodynamic factors by creating connections between the intrapsychic drives promoting maladaptive functioning and investigating with clients how these drives can be normalized toward healthy functioning. In children, this process typically occurs through the therapists' attempts to reframe problems within the theoretical model. Thus, when a child complains of test anxiety, but then reveals that the source is based on parent approval, the therapist then considers the possibility of loss of love anxiety and invites the child to also explore this possibility through either traditional talk or play-based therapy. In a talk-based approach, the therapist may suggest, "It sounds like you worry a lot about what your parents think of you. Does that worry show up anywhere else, not just on tests?" In a play-based approach, the therapist may ask the child to play a scene in which a child's parents are angry with him or her, then work to resolve the play healthily. Regardless of the modality, if the child's responses support the initial hypothesis, then the therapist's goal becomes less focused on reducing test anxiety but more on correcting loss of love anxiety, the underlying drive behind the chief complaint. If responses do not support the hypothesis, then the therapist adjusts and moves on to a different possibility within the broader etiological model, until a point of intervention is identified.

Environmental/cultural/learned factors

Whereas genetic factors highlighted interactions between amplifiers, suppressors, and biological vulnerabilities, and while psychodynamic factors focused primarily on internal amplifiers and suppressors, the third set of propagating factors focuses externally. Environment/cultural/learned factors draw attention to external current systems (both micro and macro, see Bronfenbrenner, 2004) that may influence anxiety in children. Such systems can include, but are not necessarily limited to, family, school, local, regional, ethnic, legal, etc. Media are also a significant component of the broader cultural system. Multi-volume encyclopedias could be devoted to covering the full breadth of external factors that contribute to childhood psychopathology (see, for example, the four-volume, 4656-page set edited by Cicchetti, 2016); however, I highlight below some of the more salient factors and their roles as amplifiers and suppressors in the FELT model. Although I discuss various systems individually below, none should be understood as independent, and interactive effects are likely to abound in different ways in each individual case (see Bronfenbrenner, 2004). For example, a local disaster may cause relatively little direct stress for a small child naïve to the effects of the disaster, but the family (and/or school) may react strongly to the local "panic" that might occur, which may be further exacerbated by media coverage, and so on. Thus, when considering all these systems, therapists must consider that larger systems may impact the smaller systems (and vice versa). When this occurs, the general recommendation is to focus intervention at the highest level that can be reasonably addressed through the therapeutic relationship and which is also most likely to produce the most robust, longest-lasting changes. This level usually ends up being the family or individual system, and perhaps occasionally the classroom and/or school system, as these systems can be better stabilized to resist pathologies that exist or emerge in other, larger systems.

An additional distinction that must be made with regard to environmental/cultural/learned factors is between *situational* amplifiers/suppressors and *stable* amplifiers/suppressors. Situational amplifiers/suppressors are distinct events that alter emotional states. They may include major or minor stressors, such as the death of a loved one or an upcoming test (amplifiers), or may also include calming events, such as the presence of a loved one during a specific event or playing a favorite game (suppressors). Stable amplifiers/suppressors are more robust and longer lasting. They can include trait anxiety in a parent (amplifier; Turner, Beidel, & Costello, 1987), community violence (amplifier; Martinez & Richters, 1993), or availability of a consistent, stable support (suppressor; see Spruit et al., 2020). In the FELT model, therapists are generally encouraged to focus interventions on stable amplifiers/suppressors, as these are both more controllable and more robust, leading to more sustainable changes over time, in that stable factors can be used to mitigate situational factors.

Additionally, in describing environmental/cultural/learned factors of anxiety, my goal in this book is to focus on alerting therapists to specific issues they may want to address in treatment. An in-depth overview of effective therapeutic techniques to address all these issues is beyond the scope of the book. This is especially true of family/parent factors and school factors. Therapists will need to enlist other training models to fully address these issues. In FELT, the focus instead is on the effects of these issues on a child's own Object-relational framework (see Chapter 3), which is then used to inform and better target the creation of FELT story stems (see Chapter 11).

Family

We begin our discussion of specific environmental/cultural/learned factors with the family system. To any child, the family system is integral to survival and to adequate psychological and physical development during childhood, and a number of family-based factors have been associated with increased risk of childhood anxiety. There is a firmly documented association between parental and child anxiety (Turner et al., 1987). Components of the association include genetic predispositions passed from parent to child, parental psychopathology in general, parental modeling of anxious behaviors, and other parent–child interactions (see Francis & Chorpita, 2011). Other specific parenting behaviors associated with childhood anxiety include overprotective or overly controlling parenting, rejecting parenting, and enmeshment (Bögels & Brechman-Toussaint, 2006; Negreiros & Miller, 2014). Furthermore, general exposure to adverse family interactions increases risk for developing clinical anxiety (Drake & Ginsburg, 2012).

It is important to clarify that the relationship between parenting behaviors and childhood anxiety is correlational, reciprocal, and bidirectional (Negreiros & Miller, 2014; Wei & Kendall, 2014) – that is, not only do anxious parents tend to produce anxious progeny, but anxious children tend to exacerbate parent anxiety as well. For example, in several studies, parents of anxious children are often found to be overly vigilant to neutral/ambiguous cues from children (even when the child is not their own child), rating higher levels of anxiety than do parents of non-anxious children when witnessing the same behaviors (Aschenbrand & Kendall, 2012; Barrett et al., 1996). In this manner, parenting an anxious child can sometimes lead parents to make attributional errors about whether or not a behavior is indicative of significant anxiety.

In addition to these several family-based amplifiers, there are also a number of family-based suppressors. These include, but are not limited to, supportive relationships among family members, family social support, family predictability, and clear expectations for behavior and values (O'Connell, Boat, & Warner, 2009; Quamma & Greenberg, 1994). These findings support the idea that family-based intervention is sometimes necessary to promote healthy functioning in anxious children. Based on the above-described factors, in family-based work, primary treatment goals may include stabilization of parental anxiety, increasing perceived support among family members, decreasing overall family stressors (when possible), and promoting an authoritative (warm, but firm and predictable) parenting style. It is essential to evaluate every client's family in order to ascertain any avenues where intervention is needed at the family level.

School

The school system is another major part of children's lives, and, as a result, school-related factors can significantly impact overall childhood anxiety. A series of studies by Pianta and colleagues found teacher–child relationship patterns to moderate school adjustment on multiple levels during the first years of a child's education (Pianta & Nimetz, 1991; Pianta & Steinberg, 1992; Pianta, Steinberg, & Rollins, 1995). In general, teachers who exhibited high positive affect and moderate involvement toward students yielded students who showed more positive, functional adjustment in school (and at home). Over- or under-involvement of teachers was associated with poorer functional outcomes, with students tending to become overly dependent (with over-involvement) or fall behind (with under-involvement). Also, high-anxious children were judged to be more insecure in their teacher–child relationship patterns, needing more reassurance from teachers and/or being experienced by teachers as being more "wary" of teachers. Conversely, open communication patterns among teachers and students were associated with lower levels of parent-reported childhood anxiety. These findings suggest that for some clients, intervening in the teacher–client relationship may be necessary and beneficial to their overall progress.

School is also another potential resource for perceived support during stressful events. In a study by Varni et al. (1992), children with acquired/congenital limb loss who perceived positive social support by classmates showed significantly less depression and anxiety and higher self-esteem. Similar findings have also been established in children whose parents have recently divorced (Hoyt et al., 1990). Access to peers at school is an important aspect of positive mental health.

Many childhood anxieties become more noticeable as a direct result of school-related demands. Separation anxiety, for example, by definition is likely to manifest much more clearly at school than at home. Performance or test-related anxiety may also become more prominent. For some kids, anxieties that are well-managed in the home become intensified at school. Social anxiety and selective mutism are particularly relevant examples – whereas symptoms of these disorders may go unnoticed in a comfortable family environment, they often abound outside of the home (Sharp, Sherman, & Gross, 2007). Given all of the above, intervening directly at school (usually by coordinating with school personnel, such as teachers, counselors, and administrators) should be considered a vital component of anxiety treatment in many children.

Media

Finally, the media can play a powerful role in propagating childhood anxiety. Media, including television programs, movies, new broadcasts, radio, internet, and even videogames, can both generate and exacerbate anxiety in children (Otto et al., 2007; van der Molen & Bushman, 2008). Violence displayed not only in the news but also in movies and videogames can lead to reactions such as nightmares, bed-wetting, and other symptoms similar to those of post-traumatic stress disorder (PTSD) (Otto et al., 2007). News stories about the real world can also yield a sense of helplessness and hopelessness about one's immersion in this world, leaving the child to feel anxiety at increasingly high levels (Leiner et al., 2016).

At the same time, media also appear to play a suppressive role. Certain kinds of media communicate positive psychological functioning and teach positive coping, and some of these media have been shown to reduce psycho- and behavioral-pathology in children. A study by Sanders, Montgomery, and

Brechman-Toussaint (2000) demonstrated that a 12-episode television series called "Families" was able to successfully reduce disruptive behavior problems among 2- to 8-year-old children, when compared to a control group. Similarly, one meta-analysis (Mares & Woodard, 2005) found a number of positive effects of prosocial messages communicated through television and other media, including increased positive social interactions, decreased aggression, altruism, and improved levels of stereotyping. Interestingly, the above meta-analysis specifically did not identify any one particular television program (e.g., *Sesame Street*) to be better than another. Prosocial content through any media can be effective. Additionally, some therapeutic programs capitalize on media preferences of youth and implement anxiety-targeting interventions directly through a digital media format (Khanna & Kendall, 2010). Given all of the above results, media can have a clear role in a child's response to anxiety, and clinicians are advised to leverage media when possible to focus children on positive aspects, as described above. However, clinicians should also be aware of potential negative reactions and should be prepared to address negative reactions to media when relevant.

One of the most common uses of media in FELT is the incorporation of popular media characters (both real and fictional) to fulfill certain archetypes in Play Therapy. Popular media heroes and villains are routinely used by children and by therapists to display meaningful Object representations and to direct play in meaningful directions. For example, a child may use Dementors, from the *Harry Potter* series, to represent fear and despair. An astute therapist can then be prepared to work with the child to fight Dementors using the Patronus charm, performed in key part by accessing happy memories. So, therapists can actively teach a healthy therapeutic tool (using happy memories) through these playful media references. It is often advisable, then, for therapists to work to familiarize themselves with current media tastes of children in their practice, so that they can work fluidly in that world, but also so they can understand the Object representations and archetypes that may derive from that media.

Manifest factors

The next level in our model revolves around manifest factors, which are the factors most commonly associated with the clinical symptoms of the various anxiety disorders. Whereas the propagating factors focus on managing lifetime risk of anxious functioning, manifest factors focus on managing current symptoms as they are displayed by the individual client. Manifest factors can be used to differentiate anxiety from other disorders. In the FELT model (and in research data on FELT), each of the manifest factors is believed to be present to some level in *all* clinically anxious individuals. They are categorized under two broad subtypes: biological dysfunction and negative affect. Each subtype is discussed more extensively below.

It should be noted that the manifest factors in the FELT model share many similarities with the tripartite model of anxiety and depression (Clark, Watson, & Mineka, 1994), which has garnered a tremendous amount of research and theoretical support since it was proposed. The three parts of the tripartite model include negative affect (NA), autonomic arousal (AA), and positive affect (PA). In the tripartite model, Clark and Watson suggested that a single factor, NA, was common to both anxiety and depression. The other two factors, anxious hyperarousal (high AA) and anhedonia (or low PA), differentiated anxiety from depression. In the Clark and Watson model, anxious individuals show high rates of NA and AA, while depressed individuals possessed high NA and low PA. These findings have been further supported by additional research (Barlow, 2000; Brown & Barlow, 2009). Given the above, and given that the current FELT model focuses on anxiety, but not depression, I include only NA and AA in manifest factors in this model. Although low PA is associated with some anxiety disorders (see Brown & Barlow, 2009), it is not included as a manifest factor in the FELT model. Rather, clinicians are instructed to consider low PA as a potential co-morbidity to address as needed in treatment. I also use a broader nomenclature of "biological dysfunction," rather than AA, in order to capture the irregularities that occur in both the central *and* autonomic nervous systems. Furthermore, although the tripartite model provides a strong, parsimonious baseline for understanding affective disorders, FELT includes greater specificity (rather than parsimony) so that clinicians can more specifically identify targets for intervention, as will be described in greater detail below.

Biological dysfunction

The neurobiology of anxiety is extremely complex, and, for most therapists, having a detailed understanding of the molecular neuropharmacology associated with anxiety does not have a strong direct effect on the practice of psychotherapy. Such detailed knowledge does matter in psychiatry and in medication management, but for non-prescribing therapists, it is usually sufficient to know what to expect from and when to recommend medications, and which medications may be recommended. On the other hand, a rudimentary knowledge of some of the biological cascade of stress responses, and, importantly, how to manage those behaviorally, is an essential component of psychotherapy for anxiety.

Because biological factors and neuropharmacological approaches to anxiety are detailed and complex, I present these factors on their own in Chapter 7.

Negative affect

Negative affect (NA), also commonly referred to as neuroticism (Eysenck, 1967), represents a fundamental trait that results in being high strung, nervous, or overly emotional. Individuals with high NA experience more feelings of dysphoria, worry, and irritability (Denollet, 2005). They also tend to have a negative Self-view and tend to be hypervigilant to signs of impending danger or turmoil (Watson & Pennebaker, 1989). This trait has been found to have a significant genetic component (Clark, Watson, & Mineka, 1994), with heritability estimates ranging from 30% to 50% (Barlow, 2000). NA is traditionally classified as a stable trait/temperament, which suggests NA to be a construct with stability in individuals across time and situations. This means that the set of behaviors associated with NA are expected to be displayed in a variety of situations and are believed to be a component of personality.

As a general construct, NA is useful for developing relatively parsimonious hypotheses about factors in emotional disorders. As the common factor in emotional disorders, high NA successfully differentiates anxious people from non-anxious people. However, from a treatment perspective, NA as a broad construct does little to inform clinicians about what kinds of vulnerabilities are demonstrated by high-NA individuals. In other words, although NA appears to capture a substantial portion of anxious vulnerabilities, the construct lacks the specificity necessary to inform clinicians about what cognitions, behaviors, and systemic liabilities should be targeted during treatment. Thus, in the current model, NA is broken down into four parts, each of which is targeted separately during treatment. These four parts include: anxiety sensitivity, anxiety avoidance, reduced self-efficacy, and Persistent Anxious Cognitions.

Anxiety sensitivity

Reiss et al. (1986) defined anxiety sensitivity (AS) as the belief that symptoms of anxiety will have harmful physical, psychological, or social consequences for the individual experiencing them. As a result, people with AS tend to become quite distressed by the simple presence of anxiety symptoms. When they perceive anxious symptoms, highly anxiety-sensitive people tend to engage in catastrophic misinterpretations of those symptoms, which then lead to more anxiety and, if unchecked, eventual panic. As a result, AS has been most traditionally associated in the scientific literature with panic disorder (Noël & Francis, 2011; Taylor, Cox, & Asmundson, 2009). Nonetheless, it has also shown relatively strong correlations with other anxiety symptoms in youth (Horenstein et al., 2018). Furthermore, a meta-analysis of the relevant literature found that AS reliably differentiates anxiety-disordered youth from non-clinical youth (d = 0.64, Noël & Francis, 2011). Such findings have led many scientists to believe that AS is one of the key features of pathological anxiety in youth (and adults). Consequently, AS is a primary treatment target for clinicians. A vital component of treatment becomes the task of allowing clients to experience anxiety as being tolerable and manageable.

Avoidance of anxiety: the behavioral inhibition system

Gray (1987) originally described a behavioral inhibition system (BIS) that has been linked to trait anxiety and anxiety disorders in adults and children (Kimbrel, 2009; MacAndrew & Steele, 1991; Vervoort et al., 2010). The BIS is a term used to describe a neural system that is sensitive to punishment and, as a result, organizes responses intended to avoid aversive stimuli. It is this latter function that makes the BIS important here (as sensitivity to punishment is captured under AS, described above). In order to minimize the frequency and intensity of unpleasant experiences, the BIS stimulates avoidance of those unpleasant experiences. To avoid those stimuli, a person must be able to predict how and when they might occur, which leads to vigilance. At high levels, such vigilance becomes hypervigilance, or, anxiety. In this manner, paradoxically, efforts meant to reduce anxiety about the occurrence of unpleasant stimuli lead to more anxiety (this model is described thoroughly by Borkovec, 1994). If the person experiencing that anxiety is also anxiety-sensitive, he or she will experience the very act of avoiding aversion as being aversive. Such a person is then found in a no-win situation, and anxiety increases exponentially. Thus, another major goal for clinicians is to target this behavioral inhibition and reduce anxiety avoidance. This goal, however, cannot be accomplished without first reducing AS. Only after being given an opportunity to experience anxious-like states as being tolerable and manageable can a child feel comfortable with *approaching* anxiety, instead of avoiding it. By approaching anxiety, the child activates the other system in Gray's model, the behavioral approach system (BAS), which is linked with reward and positive feelings (Gray, 1987). The goal of such an approach is to "rewire" the brain into perceiving anxiety as an adaptive emotion meant to alert a person that something in the internal or external environment needs to be solved. If anxiety is viewed as adaptive, not aversive, it can be used as a tool to promote ultimately positive outcomes. Therefore, in FELT, children are encouraged to approach anxious topics and are explicitly instructed about the adaptive nature of anxious feelings. In this manner, children come to understand anxiety as a normal emotion, that, when optimized, actually promotes positive and constructive performance (Yerkes & Dodson, 1908).

A word of caution, however, is warranted in that clinicians should be careful not to stimulate overgeneralization of the approach tactic. Children must not confuse the goal of approaching anxiety with the goal of approaching anxiety-provoking situations. Although some situations may be approachable (e.g., testing), others may be dangerous (e.g., wandering away from parents in a crowded mall). Thus, if children overgeneralize the principle of approach, they may run the risk of engaging in risky or dangerous behavior. The approach to anxiety means only that the emotion itself is sought to be understood with regard to how that emotion interacts with achieving optimal outcomes in various situations. It does *not* mean that anxiety is ignored or subjugated for the sake of achieving a certain goal (e.g., being independent from parents). The goal is to remain "in contact" with, and accept, the internal experience (see Hayes, Strosahl, & Wilson, 1999).

Reduced self-efficacy

As stated previously, individuals with high NA frequently struggle with low views about the Self. A frequent problem for anxious individuals is not only that they are anxious, but that they also feel as if they have little control over their symptoms (Barlow, 2000). Furthermore, anxious children generally engage in more negative and less positive Self-evaluations than their non-anxious cohorts (Zatz & Chassin, 1985). Thus, a key issue in the treatment of negative affectivity is to engage in measures meant to combat the sense of powerlessness that individuals are likely to feel regarding their anxiety. Clinically, the promotion of self-efficacy can occur on multiple levels and is achieved in many therapies at the individual level through the mastery of increasing levels of fear in a fear hierarchy. Additionally, clinicians may encourage self-efficacy through a broad, strengths-based approach by stimulating recognition of a child's strengths across multiple relevant realms – for example, in sports, in academics, in art, etc. – and then by working to apply those strengths directly to combatting anxiety.

Persistent Anxious Cognitions

Anxious cognitions (worry) are thought to be one of the most defining features of NA (Lawrence & Brown, 2009). Within the FELT model, anxious cognitions fall under the rubric of negative conditional logic. Statements in conditional logic are traditionally divided into two parts: the condition/antecedent (*if…* statement) and the consequent (*then…* statement). Pathological worriers frequently struggle with a narrow focus on negative consequences. In anticipating a given condition (e.g., "*if a storm occurs…*"), pathological worriers assume a negative consequent (e.g., "*…it might become a tornado.*"). The persistence of such anxious cognitions means that, more often than not, an anxious person will conclude the negative consequent, which ultimately leads to NA. A major clinical goal, then, would be to help clients more frequently entertain alternative possible consequents (e.g., "*…it might not become a tornado.*"). By habitually practicing positive conditional resolution, it is believed that children will tend to broaden their previously narrow focus on negative outcomes. As a result, the persistence of negative conditional logic is expected to fade away. In FELT, all of this is achieved through play.

Temporal factors

In a model proposed by Davidson (1998), a key emphasis in affect regulation is the issue of time (as cited in McClure & Pine, 2006). In this model, pathology is described as a perturbation in the normal, adaptive temporal sequence of emotion processing. Some disorders are characterized by disruptions that occur early in the response, while other disorders are characterized by later disruptions. By using temporal dynamics, clinicians can develop a working knowledge about when to intervene during the course of an anxious response. For example, worry occurs *before* a stimulus. Thus, potential worried thoughts should be identified and worked on prior to introduction of the anxiety-provoking stimulus. Alternatively, fear occurs *after* the stimulus. Therefore, fear responses can only be regulated after the introduction or in the presence of the feared stimulus. Some anticipatory anxiety and some reactive fear are normal for many stimuli, and sometimes these can be very intense and still within normal ranges. For example, a genuinely life-threatening event occurring in a person's near vicinity can elicit very intense feelings of fear, which would not be considered maladaptive. It is when these experiences persist beyond their normal start and stop periods that clinically significant symptoms arise.

Other temporal factors include specific vulnerabilities across development. Many of these factors were reviewed in previous chapters as we explored the development of the Self, and associated vulnerabilities, across childhood. Children also commonly experience a predictable developmental (temporal) trajectory in their anxieties. For example, young children, generally between the ages of three and six, frequently and normatively express numerous specific fears. These specific fears tend also to revolve around common triggers, including bugs, certain animals, darkness, and fictional creatures (e.g., monsters). Early childhood fears also tend to be concrete. Young children fear the dark because the dark is scary; they are rarely able to elaborate extensively on why the dark is scary, except, perhaps, to say that monsters come out at night (and monsters are scary). As children age though, around ages six to nine, their fears grow. In fact, it is during this period that childhood fears/anxieties are expected to be at their worst. This worsening occurs because during middle childhood, children develop the capacity to now imagine more realistic things that can happen to them. So, whereas young children feared the dark because of monsters, older children fear the dark because they worry, "What if someone breaks into my house and kidnaps me at night?" or, "What if a huge tornado comes and destroys my house while we're all asleep?" Advanced thinking skills, then, often translate to growing fears for children, and without healthy coping skills to manage these growing skills, children can easily become overwhelmed with anxieties. So, from a temporal perspective, clinicians should be aware that children in middle to late elementary school are expected to have greater anxieties than younger children, and that it is not uncommon for parents to report that their children's anxieties seem to worsen around this time period.

Separation anxiety also has key temporal components. Separation anxiety prior to age six is quite normal. In fact, diagnostic manuals often specify extra caution in diagnosing Separation Anxiety Disorder prior to age six, because non-clinical separation anxiety is so common in young children. Actual Separation Anxiety Disorder is also common. In fact, it is described in the *DSM-5* as being the most common anxiety disorder in children under 12. Still, like specific fears, separation anxiety changes in how it presents over time. In early childhood, it is readily recognizable. Children will show extreme distress (crying, screaming, etc.) when separated from parents, and this is very common and usually self-resolves over time. As children age, though, separation anxiety can become more subtle, manifesting as worry about a parent's health or safety and frequently checking in with them throughout the day (e.g., through phone calls or texts) seeking reassurance they are okay. Separation anxiety in older children can also manifest through fears of being kidnapped or getting lost in public places, and these worries can generate more internal distress than external distress, such that intense separation anxiety is not always obvious or clearly observable. So, clinicians assessing childhood anxiety should be alert to more subtle signs of separation fears as children age, so that persisting symptoms can be identified and managed properly.

As children move toward peri-adolescence and teenagerhood, they typically begin to develop more generalized and social fears, and they also have an increased risk for panic attacks and panic disorder. This does not mean that younger children cannot be diagnosed with generalized, social anxiety, or panic disorders; it only means that these disorders are more common during and after adolescence. So, again, another temporal factor in the assessment of anxiety is to determine if such conditions are presenting earlier than is normally expected. Often, young children with advanced cognitive ability may demonstrate worried thoughts that are more typical of older children. In such cases, younger children can have cognitive and perceptual reasoning abilities more in line with those of teenagers, and consequently their worried thoughts take on a more mature manifestation than is usually expected during the pre-adolescent/elementary stage. So, clinicians should know that temporal trends in the typical manifestations of worry across childhood do not mean that children outside those temporal trends cannot develop very similar worries.

Another temporal factor relevant to childhood anxiety comes from research into early adverse childhood experiences (ACEs) and their effects on human brain development and on other psychological outcomes. One particularly influential line of childhood trauma research has explored how ACEs impact early brain development. It is well known that the human brain grows most rapidly at two different stages of life (postnatally): from birth to age five and then again during adolescence. Early childhood brain growth is primarily concerned with developing the basic structures of the brain necessary for adaptation later in life, and by age five the human brain will have reached nearly its adult size and have all of the essential structures that the adult brain has. Adolescent brain growth, on the other hand, is more focused on solidifying connections between existing structures to help boost maturity and interconnectivity. From an evolutionary standpoint, humans have an extremely long childhood (see Konner, 2010). In fact, evolutionarily speaking, and from a brain development perspective, humans are born about 12 months earlier than they should be. Whereas in most other primates and mammals, the steep curve of brain development levels to a more gradual process at birth, in humans, that steep prenatal curve continues for about another year postnatally (see Konner, 2010). To put this another way, our closest biological animal relative, the chimpanzee, is born with a brain about half its adult size. The human brain reaches this same relative size at around 36 weeks after birth.

Why is this important? Human brains are unlike those of any other primate species in that our brains do the majority of development *outside the womb*. This means that our brains are able to adapt to our environmental surroundings better than any other primate (and perhaps better than any other animal). This is because brain development is highly experience-dependent. This does not mean that genetic endowment is not also important – it most certainly is – but the human brain, especially during the first year of life, is growing and shedding neurons at such a rapid pace in early childhood that it can actually adapt in real time to the needs of the surrounding environment. Though this idea goes against traditional evolutionary thinking – that adaptations occur slowly, over many generations – the brain is different from other organs and organisms. Throughout early childhood, brain development is doing two primary things: apoptosis and myelination. Apoptosis refers to a form of programmed (normal) cell death. At birth, humans actually have billions more neurons than they will need/use later in life, and so much of early brain development is spent *pruning* these extra neurons. Pruning is somewhat (though not completely) an experience-dependent phenomenon, following the basic principle of "if you don't use it, you lose it." In other words, the brain learns what neurons it will need and it keeps those, while neglecting the others.

Myelination is similar. Myelin is a fatty sheath that covers axons. It is the "white matter" in brains (whereas neurons are the "gray matter"). It is myelin's job to allow neurons to communicate with each other more efficiently. The metaphor I often use in teaching is to imagine an electrical wire. Myelin is like the rubber coating of the electrical wire. If you strip the coating from a wire, it no longer works as efficiently, and some of the electrical charge can "escape" through the naked, exposed part of the wire (hence why you might get shocked if you touch a live, stripped wire). Newborn and infant brains have very sparse myelin, and so their neurons don't fire very efficiently. That's also why newborns have jerky, poorly controlled movements – their brain wiring doesn't fire very well, because they lack the myelin to direct the electrical flows of their brain cells efficiently. Over the first year of life, infants develop a ton of myelin, which develops also in an experience-dependent fashion. The brain cells that the infant uses get the most attention, and thus, the most myelin.

So, when it comes to ACEs, early stressful experiences in infants, especially if they are severe and chronic, can train the infant brain to more efficiently activate stress-response neurons. In fact, this is exactly what we see in the brains of children with high levels of ACEs. Though our technology is not yet advanced enough to actually note the increased myelination of these areas, we do see on PET imaging (which shows brain activity) that children with high levels of ACEs show increased activity in specific brain areas associated with anxiety and a stress response. Furthermore, children with high levels of ACEs produce more consistently high levels of cortisol than children with more normative childhoods, another indicator that the brain has learned, through experience, to change its functioning in response to the environment.

So, temporal dynamics are important here because we know that children have an especially vulnerable period of development during the first five years of life which may predispose them to later problematic functioning. Similar ideas can be said of adolescence, when a second major neural growth spurt occurs. This growth spurt is different though because the brain is making fewer architectural changes and instead more organizational changes. I often use two metaphors here. Imagine the brain up to adolescence has been slowly collecting puzzle pieces throughout its life, and let's say it's a billion-piece puzzle where you only get a few pieces at a time, collected over 15[1] years or so. As you're collecting the pieces, you need to put them somewhere, so you fit them into the general area you think they're going to go. Where you've put each piece may not be the best place to put it, but it's "close enough" for now, because you know you're going to get more pieces later. It's not until you have all the pieces that you can really decide where that piece should go. A similar metaphor is imagining you are furnishing a mansion, and you've slowly collected furniture and decorations and everything else that goes inside for 15 years. Now that you look at it all though, you start to think, "I'm not totally happy with where I put that couch – it doesn't really go too well with the chair I bought last week." So, you move it to a better place. This is what the adolescent brain is doing, except that the brain is not literally moving neurons around (that's just not the way it works). Instead, it's just organizing connections in different ways.

As the adolescent brain is reorganizing, it is focusing primarily on higher-order brain structures – in particular, the executive functions and emotion management skills. Executive functions are still rather poorly developed in adolescence (on average, executive function reaches maturity around age 25), so adolescents really tend to struggle with organizing executive functions like planning ahead, solving problems while considering all the parts of the problem, and rapidly switching attention between complex concepts. They are also pumping out post-pubertal hormones, which give them a new range of drives and emotions they never experienced before, which they must now reorganize into the brain. This will take years to get it "right," but eventually, most teens succeed in this reorganizational process and are able to reach heightened maturity in their abilities to connect ideas, drives, emotions, and other needs.

So, similarly to how children experience biological vulnerabilities during the first five years of life, they experience a second surge of vulnerability at adolescence. Unhealthy organizational adaptations that occur during adolescence, then, tend to become more solidified and resistant to change if not addressed during the critical developmental period. This does not mean that the brain is in a permanent, unchangeable state after adolescence. Quite the opposite, in fact; adults can benefit from psychotherapy too. Rather, it only means that adult psychotherapy must commonly address and "reprogram" psychological malalignments that occurred during childhood and adolescence. If we can intervene instead during or before these vulnerable stages, we help predispose these youth to grow into psychologically more flexible and healthier adults.

What does all this mean for FELT?

Now that we've seen the FELT etiological model, we must now integrate that model into what a therapist actually does in psychotherapy. For this, let us return to the figure of the FELT etiological model, Figure 6.1 (on page 99).

First, FELT clinicians must simultaneously attend to and intervene across all three levels of the etiological model. It is insufficient to simply focus on manifest symptoms of anxiety. Rather, clinicians must also address the propagating factors relevant to each individual client, at least as much as is possible. Obviously, the exception to this is genetics, as psychotherapists do not target genes through therapy. Still, they can focus on maximizing suppressors (of genetic risks) and minimizing amplifiers, as described in detail throughout this chapter. Environmental intervention is most commonly accomplished through coordination with parents/caregivers to help correct any factors there that may amplify anxiety risk. Occasionally, environmental intervention involves coordination with schools as well, when this seems necessary. Environmental factors also influence the formation of a child's internal Object-relations, so these must be considered within each client's Object-relational case conceptualization. Psychodynamic factors are a main focus of individual therapy, with therapists working to identify which basic human needs contribute to each individual client's manifest anxiety, and then working to help resolve these needs in healthy ways.

Manifest factors are then managed through teaching coping skills. Again, biological dysfunction and its associated pharmacological and behavioral interventions are covered in the next chapter. NA is addressed by focusing on four subfactors. Specifically, therapists address the four subfactors of NA by instead teaching their opposites. In lieu of AS, therapists move children toward anxiety tolerance. Instead of anxiety avoidance, therapists promote anxiety approach. Therapists also build children's self-efficacy and intervene to control the persistence of anxious cognitions. Furthermore, in my experience with childhood anxiety, all children with clinically significant anxiety experience all the manifest factors, at least to some extent. The same cannot be said of propagating factors, which are different for each child, and thus, therapists have more flexibility in individualizing treatment of propagating factors. However, with manifest factors, therapeutic goals/targets are consistent across all clinically anxious children.

Lastly, temporal factors are rarely addressed directly in psychotherapy. Instead, therapists simply use temporal information to help choose/prioritize specific targets for therapy. For example, if presented with a clinically anxious four-year-old whose biological parents' rights were recently terminated due to severe neglect, a therapist may choose to focus much more heavily on environmental factors in this case, rather than on individual factors, helping work to secure placement in a permanent loving home, and then working on attachment to these new caregivers. In this case, the temporal vulnerabilities of the child needing to form secure attachments before age five would take precedence over the manifest anxiety that presents due to the disrupted attachments. This does not mean the therapist could not simultaneously work to teach anxiety management skills too, but their primary focus would be to do so through an attachment-focused lens, hoping to start as soon as possible the corrective process of this child's early brain development. The therapist could still achieve this work within the FELT etiological model, especially following some of the Object-relational needs of the child as they work together, but the execution of intervention in FELT would likely need to be changed to accommodate neglect-related needs, incorporating other evidence-based models better tested with children with histories of neglect.

Note

1 This is an arbitrary number for the purposes of the illustration. It should not be implied that the adolescent brain growth spurt necessarily occurs at age 15.

REFERENCES

Aschenbrand, S. G., & Kendall, P. C. (2012). The effect of perceived child anxiety status on parental latency to intervene with anxious and nonanxious youth. *Journal of Consulting and Clinical Psychology*, 80(2), 232–238.

Barlow, D. H. (2000). Unraveling the mysteries of anxiety and its disorders from the perspective of emotion theory. *American Psychologist*, 55(11), 1247–1263.

Barrett, P. M., Dadds, M. R., Rapee, R. M., & Ryan, S. M. (1996). Family enhancement of cognitive style in anxious and aggressive children. *Journal of Abnormal Child Psychology*, 24(2), 187–203.

Bögels, S. M., & Brechman-Toussaint, M. L. (2006). Family issues in child anxiety: attachment, family functioning, parental rearing and beliefs. *Clinical Psychology Review*, 26(7), 834–856.

Borkovec, T. D. (1994). The nature, functions, and origins of worry. In G. C. L. Davey & F. Tallis (Eds.), *Worrying: Perspectives on Theory, Assessment and Treatment* (pp. 5–33). Hoboken, NJ: John Wiley & Sons.

Bronfenbrenner, U. (Ed.). (2004). *Making Human Beings Human: Bioecological Perspectives on Human Development*. Thousand Oaks, CA: Sage Publications.

Brown, T. A., & Barlow, D. H. (2009). A proposal for a dimensional classification system based on the shared features of the *DSM-IV* anxiety and mood disorders: implications for assessment and treatment. *Psychological Assessment*, 21(3), 256–271.

Carmichael, A. (1990). Physical development and biological influences. In B. Tonge, G. D. Burrows, & J. S. Werry (Eds.), *Handbook of Studies in Child Psychiatry* (pp. 119–136). Amsterdam: Elsevier.

Cicchetti, D. (2016). *Developmental Psychopathology* (4 vols., 3rd ed.). Hoboken, NJ: Wiley.

Clark, L. A., Watson, D., & Mineka, S. (1994). Temperament, personality, and the mood and anxiety disorders. *Journal of Abnormal Psychology*, 103(1), 103–116.

Costa, P. T., & McCrae, R. R. (1987). Validation of the five-factor model of personality across instruments and observers. *Journal of Personality and Social Psychology*, 52(1), 81–90.

Denollet, J. (2005). DS14: standard assessment of negative affectivity, social inhibition, and Type D personality. *Psychosomatic Medicine*, 67(1), 89–97.

Drake, K. L., & Ginsburg, G. S. (2012). Family factors in the development, treatment, and prevention of childhood anxiety disorders. *Clinical Child and Family Psychology Review*, 15 (2), 144–162.

Eysenck, H. J. (1967). *The Biological Basis of Personality*. Springfield, IL: C. C. Thomas.

Francis, S. E., & Chorpita, B. F. (2011). Parental beliefs about child anxiety as a mediator of parent and child anxiety. *Cognitive Therapy and Research*, 35(1), 21–29.

Gabbard, G. (2014). *Psychodynamic Psychiatry in Clinical Practice* (5th ed.). Arlington, VA: American Psychiatric Publishing, Inc.

Giedd, J. N., Snell, J. W., Lange, N., Rajapakse, J. C., Casey, B. J., Kozuch, P. L., ... & Rapoport, J. L. (1996). Quantitative magnetic resonance imaging of human brain development: ages 4–18. *Cerebral Cortex*, 6(4), 551–559.

Göttken, T., White, L. O., Klein, A. M., & von Klitzing, K. (2014). Short-term psychoanalytic child therapy for anxious children: a pilot study. *Psychotherapy*, 51(1), 148–158.

Gray, J. A. (1987). Perspectives on anxiety and impulsivity: a commentary. *Journal of Research in Personality*, 21(4), 493–509.

Guzowski, J. F., Setlow, B., Wagner, E. K., & McGaugh, J. L. (2001). Experience-dependent gene expression in the rat hippocampus after spatial learning: a comparison of the immediate-early genes *Arc*, c-*fos*, and *zif268*. *The Journal of Neuroscience*, 21(14), 5089–5098.

Hamadeh, H. K., Bushel, P. R., Jayadev, S., Martin, K., DiSorbo, O., Sieber, S., ... & Afshari, C. A. (2002). Gene expression analysis reveals chemical-specific profiles. *Toxicological Sciences*, 67(2), 219–231.

Harter, S. (2012). *The Construction of the Self: Developmental and Sociocultural Foundations* (2nd ed.). New York: Guilford.

Hayes, S. C., Strosahl, K. D., & Wilson, K. G. (1999). *Acceptance and Commitment Therapy: An Experiential Approach to Behavior Change*. New York: Guilford.

Horenstein, A., Potter, C. M., & Heimberg, R. G. (2018). How does anxiety sensitivity increase risk of chronic medical conditions? *Clinical Psychology: Science and Practice*, 25(3), e12248.

Hoyt, L. A., Cowen, E. L., Pedro-Carroll, J. L., & Alpert-Gillis, L. J. (1990). Anxiety and depression in young children of divorce. *Journal of Clinical Child Psychology*, 19(1), 26–32.

Issa, J. P. (2000). CpG-island methylation in aging and cancer. *Current Topics in Microbiology and Immunology*, 249, 101–118.

Khanna, M. S., & Kendall, P. C. (2010). Computer-assisted cognitive behavioral therapy for child anxiety: results of a randomized clinical trial. *Journal of Consulting and Clinical Psychology*, 78(5), 737–745.

Kimbrel, N. (2009). *BIS, BAS, and Bias: The Role of Personality and Cognition in Social Anxiety* [Doctoral dissertation, University of North Carolina, Greenville]. https://libres.uncg.edu/ir/uncg/f/Kimbrel_uncg_0154D_10099.pdf.

Konner, M. (2010). *The Evolution of Childhood: Relationships, Emotion, Mind*. Cambridge, MA: Harvard University Press.

Lawrence, A. E., & Brown, T. A. (2009). Differentiating generalized anxiety disorder from anxiety disorder not otherwise specified. *The Journal of Nervous and Mental Disease*, 197(12), 879–886.

Leiner, M., Peinado, J., Villanos, M. T., Lopez, I., Uribe, R., & Pathak, I. (2016). Mental and emotional health of children exposed to news media of threats and acts of terrorism: the cumulative and pervasive effects. *Frontiers in Pediatrics*, 4, 26.

MacAndrew, C., & Steele, T. (1991). Gray's behavioral inhibition system: a psychometric examination. *Personality and Individual Differences*, 12(2), 157–171.

Mares, M.-L., & Woodard, E. (2005). Positive effects of television on children's social interactions: a meta-analysis. *Media Psychology*, 7(3), 301–322.

Martinez, P., & Richters, J. E. (1993). The NIMH community violence project: II. Children's distress symptoms associated with violence exposure. *Psychiatry*, 56(1), 22–35.

McClure, E. B., & Pine, D. S. (2006). Social anxiety and emotion regulation: a model for developmental psychopathology perspectives on anxiety disorders. In D. Cicchetti & D. J. Cohen (Eds.), *Developmental Psychopathology: Risk, Disorder, and Adaptation* (pp. 470–502). Hoboken, NJ: Wiley.

Meaney, M. (2010). Epigenetics and the biological definition of gene × environment interactions. *Child Development*, 81(1), 41–79.

Milrod, B., Shapiro, T., Gross, C., Silver, G., Preter, S., Libow, A., & Leon, A. C. (2013). Does manualized psychodynamic psychotherapy have an impact on youth anxiety disorders? *American Journal of Psychotherapy*, 67(4), 359–366.

Negreiros, J., & Miller, L. D. (2014). The role of parenting in childhood anxiety: etiological factors and treatment implications. *Clinical Psychology: Science and Practice*, 21(1), 3–17.

Noël, V. A., & Francis, S. E. (2011). A meta-analytic review of the role of child anxiety sensitivity in child anxiety. *Journal of Abnormal Child Psychology*, 39(5), 721–733.

O'Connell, M. E., Boat, T., & Warner, K. E. (2009). *Preventing Mental, Emotional, and Behavioral Disorders among Young People: Progress and Possibilities*. Washington, DC: The National Academies Press.

Otto, M. W., Henin, A., Hishfeld-Becker, D. R., Pollack, M. H., Biederman, J., & Rosenbaum, J. F. (2007). Posttraumatic stress disorder symptoms following media exposure to tragic events: impact of 9/11 on children at risk for anxiety disorders. *Journal of Anxiety Disorders*, 21(7), 888–902.

Parsch, J., & Ellegren, H. (2013). The evolutionary causes and consequences of sex-biased gene expression. *Nature Reviews Genetics*, 14(2), 83–87.

Pfefferbaum, A., Mathalon, D. H., Sullivan, E. V., Rawles, J. M., Zipursky, R. B., & Iim, K. O. (1994). A quantitative magnetic resonance imaging study of changes in brain morphology from infancy to late adulthood. *Archives of Neurology*, 51(9), 874–887.

Pianta, R. C., & Nimetz, S. L. (1991). Relationships between children and teachers: associations with home and classroom behavior. *Journal of Applied Developmental Psychology*, 12(3), 379–393.

Pianta, R. C., & Steinberg, M. (1992). Teacher-child relationships and the process of adjusting to school. *New Directions for Child Development*, 57, 61–80.

Pianta, R. C., Steinberg, M. S., & Rollins, K. B. (1995). The first two years of school: teacher-child relationships and deflections in children's classroom adjustment. *Development and Psychopathology*, 7(2), 295–312.

Quamma, J. P., & Greenberg, M. T. (1994). Children's experience of life stress: the role of family social support and social problem-solving skills as protective factors. *Journal of Clinical Child Psychology*, 23(3), 295–305.

Reik, W., & Walter, J. (2001). Genomic imprinting: parental influence on the genome. *Nature Reviews Genetics*, 2(1), 21–32.

Reiss, S., Peterson, R. A., Gursky, D. M., & McNally, R. J. (1986). Anxiety sensitivity, anxiety frequency and the prediction of fearfulness. *Behaviour Research and Therapy*, 24(1), 1–8.

Sanders, M. R., Montgomery, D. T., & Brechman-Touissant, M. L. (2000). The mass media and the prevention of child behavior problems: the evaluation of a television series to promote positive outcomes for parents and their children. *Journal of Child Psychology & Psychiatry*, 41(7), 939–948.

Sharp, W. G., Sherman, C., & Gross, A. M. (2007). Selective mutism and anxiety: a review of the current conceptualization of the disorder. *Journal of Anxiety Disorders*, 21(4), 568–579.

Siegel, D. J. (2020). *The Developing Mind: How Relationships and the Brain Interact to Shape Who We Are* (3rd ed.). New York: Guilford.

Silverman, W. A. (2004). A cautionary tale about supplemental oxygen: The albatross of neonatal medicine. *Pediatrics*, 113(2), 394–396.

Spruit, A., Goos, L., Weenink, N., Rodenburg, R., Niemeyer, H., Stams, G. J., & Colonnesi, C. (2020). The relation between attachment and depression in children and adolescents: a multilevel meta-analysis. *Clinical Child and Family Psychology Review*, 23(1), 54–69.

Sturtevant, A. H. (1913). The Himalayan rabbit case, with some considerations on multiple allelomorphs. *American Naturalist*, XLVII(556), 234–239.

Szyf, M. (2009). Early life, the epigenome and human health. *Acta Paediatrica*, 98(7), 1082–1084.

Taylor, S., Cox, B. J., & Asmundson, G. J. G. (2009). Anxiety disorders: panic and phobias. In P. H. Blaney & T. Millon (Eds.), *Oxford Textbook of Psychopathology* (pp. 120–145). Oxford: Oxford University Press.

Turner, S. M., Beidel, D. C., & Costello, A. (1987). Psychopathology in the offspring of anxiety disorders patients. *Journal of Consulting and Clinical Psychology*, 55(2), 229–235.

van der Molen, J. H., & Bushman, B. J. (2008). Children's direct fright and worry reactions to violence in fiction and news television programs. *Journal of Pediatrics*, 153(3), 420–424.

Varni, J. W., Setoguchi, Y., Rappaport, L. R., & Talbot, D. (1992). Psychological adjustment and perceived social support in children with congenital/acquired limb deficiencies. *Journal of Behavioural Medicine*, 15(1), 31–44.

Vervoort, L., Wolters, L. H., Hogendoorn, S. M., de Haan, E., Boer, F., & Prins, P. J. M. (2010). Sensitivity of Gray's Behavioral Inhibition System in clinically anxious and non-anxious children and adolescents. *Personality and Individual Differences*, 48(5), 629–633.

Watson, D., & Clark, L. A. (1984). Negative affectivity: the disposition to experience aversive emotional states. *Psychological Bulletin*, 96(3), 465–490.

Watson, D., & Pennebaker, J. W. (1989). Health complaints, stress, and distress: exploring the central role of negative affectivity. *Psychological Review*, 96(2), 234–254.

Wei, C., & Kendall, P. C. (2014). Child perceived parenting behavior: childhood anxiety and related symptoms. *Child & Family Behavior Therapy*, 36(1), 1–18.

Yerkes, R. M., & Dodson, J. D. (1908). The relation of strength of stimulus to rapidity of habit formation. *Journal of Comparative Neurology & Psychology*, 18(5), 459–482.

Zatz, S., & Chassin, L. (1985). Cognitions of test-anxious children under naturalistic test-taking conditions. *Journal of Consulting and Clinical Psychology*, 53(3), 393–401.

Chapter 7

Pharmacology and biological factors of childhood anxiety

In this chapter, I use some concepts of neuropharmacology to outline relevant biological factors in the etiology and manifestation of childhood anxiety. To help focus this book primarily on *psychotherapeutic* approaches to treatment, pharmacological review will be intentionally cursory, which therapists may use to educate parents and patients about when to consider medications and what to expect from them. I will also focus pharmacological review on some of the neurochemical components that can be useful for therapists. In other words, some therapeutic techniques/recommendations for anxiety can be understood as behavioral means to mimic the physiological effects offered by anxiolytic and antidepressant medication. By understanding how medications work, and what neurochemical components are targeted by medications, therapists can capitalize on their biochemical knowledge to specifically identify behavioral and psychological interventions that may address, at least to some degree, those same targets.[1]

Pharmacological approaches to anxiety treatment

FELT has been most heavily tested with children ages 4–11 (see Steadman, 2016). Thus, in discussing medications, it is important to focus on medications that are most likely to be used in early childhood. In current clinical practice, there are really three types of medications routinely used in children for managing anxiety: antihistamines, antidepressants, and (in adolescents, mainly), the azaspirodecanediane, BuSpar (buspirone, though I will not discuss buspirone below, as it is not widely used for younger children). There are other medications on the market that may be prescribed in specific situations for childhood anxiety, namely benzodiazepines, but these are not routinely used for long-term anxiety, nor should they be, as their long-term use has been shown to cause dependence and thus actually worsen anxiety over time, especially once withdrawn. Instead, benzodiazepines are typically used in hospital settings for effective, but short-term, reductions in procedure-related anxiety (i.e., prior to surgery). Still, understanding their effects can be instructive for therapists practicing with anxious children.

DOI: 10.4324/9781032693187-8

What are the clinical targets of medications used to treat anxiety?

Fulfillment. The complete neuropharmacology of anxiety is quite complex, and to properly prescribe or make prescription recommendations for medications requires advanced pharmacological training. Still, there are some key ideas that can be useful to non-prescribing therapists. First, therapists should be aware of the differences between *agonists* and *antagonists*. All drugs work through some sort of molecular binding. The drug binds to a naturally occurring chemical or receptor, which can then either block that chemical/receptor from doing what it is naturally supposed to do (antagonist), or it can cause that chemical or receptor to act when it otherwise would not (agonist). The most commonly prescribed drugs used to treat anxiety and depression are selective serotonin reuptake inhibitors (SSRIs), and, usually only if SSRIs do not sufficiently work, serotonin-norepinephrine reuptake inhibitors (SNRIs). Both of these drugs work through primarily antagonistic pathways. They block a protein that normally acts as a recycler, specifically, the serotonin transporter protein, in the case of both SSRIs and SNRIs (SNRIs block that protein *and* the norepinephrine transporter protein). Thus, SSRIs do not increase serotonin; they simply allow the body an opportunity to better use what it already has.

Imagine you've ordered a package from your favorite online store. You've been waiting for this package with great anticipation. You know that as soon as you open it, you're going to feel a great happiness. Now, let's say the post office delivered that package while you were away. It's right there on the porch, waiting for you, and you'll pick it up as soon as you've got a chance. You've got to pick up a lot of other things first, but you'll get to it when you can. Now, let's also imagine you've got a lovely, though perhaps at times overzealous neighborhood clean-up crew who picks up spare trash they see in the neighborhood. Let's say that one of the members of that crew has a job specifically to clean up cardboard boxes. If the box is in good shape, they don't throw it away. Instead, they bring it back to the post office, so the post can use it to package up other materials. The neighbor sees your box on your porch, gets a little excited, and decides to clean it up. It's in good shape, so they bring it back to the post office.

Later, you come home to open your much-expected package, but it's not there. Suddenly, your expectation for happiness has turned to dread, maybe a mixture of sadness, worry, and anger. The package was going to make your day, but you didn't get it. You can see on your security camera what happened – the cardboard-cleaning neighbor picked it up with everything else. You call the post office and tell them to redeliver the package tomorrow, and they find the package and agree to do so. Meanwhile, you visit your neighbor and give them a giant pile of carboard-like trash. It's not real cardboard; it's a fake kind, but the neighbor really likes it. They can't tell the difference, and they'll take it. Now, your neighbor's hands are too full recycling your fake cardboard for them to take your package again, even if they wanted to. Your package will stay safe and sound on your porch until you can pick it up and feel the happiness it brings.

SSRIs and SNRIs work just the same way. In the metaphor, the package is serotonin (or, in the case of SNRIs, both serotonin and norepinephrine), the neighbor is the associated transporter protein, and the fake cardboard you're offering are the SSRIs/SNRIs themselves. The post office represents your neurons, you are the receptor. Normally, your neurons will deliver serotonin and/or norepinephrine into the synapse – the gap between one neuron and another. Inside that synapse, each chemical lingers until it either connects with a receptor (in the metaphor, until it's "received" by you) or is recycled by the transporter protein or eliminated/trashed by an enzyme (this elimination is done by a different protein – monamaine oxidase (MAO) – which is how some older antidepressants (MAOIs) work, by blocking the trash collector[2]). So, leaving transmitters in the synapse longer gives them a better chance to be received by you.

This metaphor of antagonism can be quite useful in psychotherapy. It can be a used in a play scene as a way to inform children, in kid-friendly language, about how their medication works, if they are taking an SSRI or SNRI, and the metaphor can be adapted as needed for different children (e.g., the post office can be replaced by Santa Claus/Father Christmas, and the package replaced by a gift, and the neighbor replaced by the Grinch). The metaphor can also be used to explore how children respond when they do not receive something they expected. Do they respond through disappointment and "giving up," or do they work through it and either figure out a way to get what they want/need or figure out how to move forward without that thing and still find happiness? In other words, how do they seek fulfillment?

This is the lesson that biochemistry teaches us. **One major clinical target of medications is fulfillment.** Anxiety, depression, and other negative affect result at least partially from a lack of fulfillment, and healing from negative affect is much more difficult if someone continues with a lack of fulfillment. Medications like SSRIs and SNRIs do help fulfill biological needs in a very real, dependable way. However, they are not the only means toward fulfillment, and they are rarely sufficient, on their own, to lead children (or adults too, for that matter) to build the necessary behavioral, mental, and emotional skills to satisfy that psychological need for fulfillment.[3] This is where psychotherapy helps where medication cannot – skill building for long-term maintenance of gains.

Still, a sense of fulfillment is extremely unlikely if a person's biochemistry doesn't work optimally. This is where medications help. I will often talk to parents and clients about medication if a child seems, after a fair trial of good psychotherapy, unable to make progress due to being "frozen" by too much negative affect (or lack of positive affect). Medications can be an effective means to temper down negative affect or to return enough positive affect to allow a child to benefit more fully from psychotherapy, and SSRIs/SNRIs seem to be, right now, the best balance between safety and long-term efficacy for achieving this goal.

Sedation/de-arousal. Another commonly prescribed medication for anxiety is hydroxyzine. The antihistamine hydroxyzine (Atarax, Vistaril) is an H1-receptor **inverse agonist** with low to moderate antihistaminic properties. Inverse agonists are slightly different than antagonists. Inverse agonists do everything an antagonist does – blocking the site from natural (or other) agonists – but they also prevent spontaneous activity of the receptor. Some hormone receptors (histamine, being a relevant example) are partially active even without anything bound to the receptor. Inverse agonists (like anti-histamines) selectively bind to the "inactive" state of these receptors, and then lock the receptors in that inactive state. Thus, histamine receptors cannot become active as long as they are bound to an antihistamine.

Still, not all antihistamines seem to be useful in treating anxiety. Cetirizine (Zyrtec) is actually a direct metabolite of hydroxyzine – the human body converts hydroxyzine into cetirizine, and cetirizine is probably responsible for quite a bit of hydroxyzine's antihistamine effect (Gengo et al., 1987) – but cetirizine does not have the same anti-anxiety effects as hydroxyzine. Hydroxyzine is the only antihistamine with FDA approval for treating anxiety. Current clinical consensus is that hydroxyzine's sedative effects are probably most responsible for its use in treating anxiety. Hydroxyzine tempers the physiological arousal that occurs in anxiety, making the anxiety as a whole feel less intense and more manageable. However, the effects are short-lived. Onset of efficacy is usually within 15–60 minutes, and sedation normally lasts 4–6 hours, after which the potential for anxiety returns to normal. In reality, what this means is that after the arousal of an anxiety-provoking situation has passed, patients are usually left feeling sleepy. Consequently, hydroxyzine is not ideal for managing long-term, chronic anxiety. It is better for temporary relief, for example, in pediatric procedures (e.g., the dentist) where full sedation is not desirable or necessary.

Still, hydroxyzine is weak. Occasionally, prescribers need a very strong anxiolytic and sedative. This is where benzodiazepines come in. Although clinicians should not expect to see children taking benzodiazepines for managing chronic anxiety, their mechanism of action can be informative for understanding the neurobiology of anxiety and relaxation. Gamma-amino-butyric acid, better known as GABA, is the major inhibitory neuro-transmitter of the brain. In other words, the brain uses GABA to stop neurons from firing. Consequently, GABAergic drugs are extremely effective for treating any condition in which you want to stop cells from firing – most commonly, for seizures, acute anxiety, or insomnia.

Of the two main groups of GABA receptors: $GABA_A$ and $GABA_B$, $GABA_A$ is more important for understanding anxiety. The $GABA_A$ receptor was first discovered in the 1970s, when researchers explored the alkaloid bicuculline, which is found in some toxic plants, namely *Dicentra cucullaria*

(Dutchman's britches) and *Adlumia fungosa* (Allegheny vine). In other words, scientists discovered the GABA receptors by studying poisonous plants. Ingestion of bicuculline causes convulsions, and it does this by acting as an antagonist on $GABA_A$. Pentylenetetrazol is another drug that antagonizes the $GABA_A$ receptor. Though its use in most of the world has died out with better scientific advances, pentylenetetrazol was originally used in the 1930s as a form of convulsive therapy for depression. In this way, it is similar to electroconvulsive therapy (ECT) for severe, intractable depression, though ECT is now preferred as one can achieve much more precise seizure control with ECT.[4] Lastly, the extremely toxic picrotoxin, derived from the Southeast Asian fruit *Anamirta cocculus*, known in English as the Indian berry or fishberry, also affects $GABA_A$ and causes convulsions if ingested.

Shortly after the discovery that these historic toxins/drugs caused convulsions through $GABA_A$ antagonism, agonists and inverse $GABA_A$ agonists began to be developed. These drugs are called benzodiazepines, and the specific site on the $GABA_A$ receptor to which they bind is commonly called the "benzodiazepine site." Agonists at the benzodiazepine site include diazepam, lorazepam, alprazolam, and clonazepam, and they all essentially work by increasing the affinity for GABA itself at the site. There are also some partial GABA agonists, but these are not widely used outside of research. Two examples are zopiclone and pagoclone, both of which were investigated as sedatives and/or anxiolytic agents, but neither is commercially available. Zolpidem (Ambien) is a related drug that also binds to the benzodiazepine site of the $GABA_A$ receptor, but it is classified as a full agonist.

Anyone who has ever taken these drugs (usually before a procedure) will tell you they flat out work! Benzodiazepine agonists are extremely effective at practically eliminating anxiety, and they work quickly. They also cause extreme sedation. One reason you won't be anxious is because you will be asleep, especially at higher doses. Benzodiazepines ($GABA_A$ agonists) are most commonly used in hospital settings to address acute anxiety and as preoperative sedatives (in addition to barbiturates). There are prescription $GABA_A$ antagonists too, which offer more dosage control than the plant-based $GABA_A$ antagonists discussed above. Flumenazil is an example, and flumenazil can be used post-operatively to help patients "awake" from sedation caused by $GABA_A$ agonists.

So, clinically, **the primary target for both hydroxyzine and benzodiazepines is sedation**. In both cases, sedation overrides the natural physiological arousal that occurs in anxiety. The problem, of course, is that both hydroxyzine and benzodiazepines have potentially nasty side effects, including, most potently, oversedation and dependence. Anxiolytic dependence is particularly problematic because anxiolytic withdrawal is associated with very intense, worse-than-baseline anxiety. So, due to physiological dependence, long term, sedative anxiolytics actually appear to worsen anxiety, rather than improve it. These drugs can also raise a person's anxiety sensitivity.

Rather than becoming desensitized to anxiety and to anxiety-provoking stimuli, they become hypersensitive to all kinds of stress.

Stress exposure contains important lessons. It is through stress exposure that we learn we can handle stress. So, we *need* stress exposure, but we can only use stress therapeutically if we have the tools to address it, and we can really only build confidence in those tools through controlled stress exposure. If we spend our lives avoiding distress, we never fully develop our stress management tools. The lesson we learn from anxiolytics, then, is that there is a balance to be achieved between stress relaxation and complete stress avoidance. With too much sedation, you achieve stress avoidance, and with too much stress avoidance, you only worsen your long-term reactions to other stress.

So, the main psychotherapeutic lesson from sedative anxiolytics is that therapists must strike a similar balance. **We want children to be relieved of overly intense distress in the face of stressors, but we don't want them to miss stressors altogether**. Hence, when a therapist focuses on teaching relaxation skills, they also want to make sure a child client is still engaged enough to attend to and endure the exposure to stressors. It is important for us to teach children how to relax themselves – how to mimic (at a low level) the sedation achieved by hydroxyzine or even by benzodiazepines. It is equally important that these relaxation skills are then used while simultaneously attending to stressors.

In FELT, most exposures are generated through play, hence the term "Fantasy-Exposure." As emphasized previously, children experience these fantasy exposures in a very real way, but they can still tell the difference between a fantasy exposure and a real exposure. The distress caused by the Robber stem is going to be considerably less than any distress caused by actual robbers breaking into the child's home. Still, they are being exposed to therapeutic stressors, which they must learn to manage. Through healthy resolution of play, they learn to decrease anxiety sensitivity, to approach anxiety (rather than avoid it), and they build self-confidence that they can face other stressors when they need to.

In FELT, therapists also work explicitly to teach children evidence-based relaxation skills, which mimics the sedative effects of drugs, but without the risk dependence and other negative side effects that come from those drugs. The goal of relaxation training is similar to that achieved by drugs, to counter the physiological arousal of anxiety. So, in planning effective relaxation techniques, it helps for therapists not only to keep in mind the balance described above but also to understand the human body's physiological reaction to stress/anxiety.

Physiological arousal and distress in anxious humans

Anxiety tends to produce a rather predictable cascade of hormonal action within the human body. These hormones, in turn, also produce predictable physiological symptoms. In this section, we review those symptoms and how FELT therapists may manage them through Play Therapy.

Hypothalamic-pituitary-adrenal axis. One of the best-understood pheno-types of anxious people is fear, due to the ability of scientists to create and study animal models of fear. A state of fear is characterized by activation of the hypothalamic-pituitary-adrenal (HPA) axis (see Nestler, Hyman, & Malenka, 2009). When activated, the HPA axis ultimately releases the hor-mone cortisol into the bloodstream, which causes the body to enter a cata-bolic state, suppressing inflammatory responses and heightening autonomic arousal. Such autonomic arousal is characterized most prominently by vasoconstriction and increased need for oxygen (which cause increased heart rate, increased blood pressure, and heavier breathing). Other associated autonomic responses include sweating, muscle tension, gut motility/dis-rupted digestion, and diuresis (Parker et al., 2003). To stimulate the release of cortisol from the adrenal gland in humans, the hypothalamus begins by releasing corticotrophin-releasing factor (CRF), which communicates with the pituitary gland to release adrenocorticotropic hormone (ACTH), which finally communicates with the adrenal gland to release cortisol. CRF is important because it also serves as a neurotransmitter and is received by neurons in the central nucleus of the amygdala, which then projects to other areas of the brain to activate other fear responses including pain suppres-sion, defensive behavioral responses (i.e., behavioral freezing), enhanced vigilance, and the formation of memories about the conditions under which the danger has occurred. Projections from the amygdala also allow humans to identify the subjective experience of fear ("I am afraid!") and plan the appropriate response. These normal fear responses are all adaptive for sur-vival, and are thus hardwired, to some extent, in every human being on the planet; however, individual differences regarding both automatic and plan-ned fear responses do exist, and individuals whose responses approach or reach the extreme end of the spectrum are those who are most susceptible to pathological anxiety.

Individuals with excessive anxiety exhibit abnormal autonomic arousal (e.g., excessive or prolonged arousal), maladaptive behavioral and cognitive respon-ses, and overly generalized or poorly specified memory activation and encoding (see Nestler, Hyman, & Malenka, 2009). Thus, during acute cortisol release in response to anxiety-provoking situations, excessively anxious persons may phy-siologically show panic (heart racing, shortness of breath, sweating) and/or they may show more subtle effects, such as muscle soreness/tightness, headaches, or stomach aches. Behaviorally, they may find themselves "keyed up," as a "fight" response; may avoid situations, as a "flee" response; or may become indecisive and stuck, as in a "freeze" response. With excessively anxious individuals, such responding occurs even in the absence of an objective threat or danger. Thus, biologically and cognitively, they often perceive threats in situations where others do not. In these situations, the HPA axis responds just the same. Therefore, one key area of intervention for clinicians treating anxiety is to help regulate the HPA axis.

HPA downregulation, though, is actually seen as a negative side effect of several drugs, and this is especially undesirable in children, as the HPA axis is also responsible for growth hormone release, thyroid hormone release, and vasopression (or antidiuretic hormone), all of which are essential for optimal healthy functioning. Chronic corticosteroid use is generally avoided for these reasons, because corticosteroid use (such as prednisone, prednisolone) is well known to cause HPA suppression. HPA suppression is another reason patients must taper off high-dose corticosteroids. Rapid withdrawal of corticosteroids can essentially strip the body of cortisol and HPA activity, which can lead to feelings of severe fatigue, malaise, fever, joint aches, and other flu-like symptoms. It can also leave the body incapable of responding to stress, which can cause a crisis if, for example, a person must enter surgery immediately after abrupt withdrawal of steroids. Consequently, chemical HPA downregulation is not currently a target of therapeutic action of any anxiolytic drugs, simply because its effects on the body are too widespread and too interlinked.

Behavioral HPA downregulation (toward healthy levels), though, can be promoted through psychotherapy, and this is supported by some psychotherapy research, especially in the area of childhood trauma. Children who have experienced chronic stress, such as through long-term trauma, have been shown to have irregular cortisol levels (Laurent et al., 2015). Rather than follow the typical diurnal schedule of cortisol, which is highest in the morning and decreases slowly over the course of the day, children with chronic (years long) trauma/stress show consistently high cortisol levels throughout the day. Therapy studies that have investigated changes in children who have received long-term treatment for trauma/chronic stress show that behavioral techniques and important environmental changes (i.e., removing children from the trauma) can actually normalize that cortisol function, such that it eventually moves toward (and perhaps even reaches) the healthy standard (Castro-Vale & Carvalho, 2020). So, psychotherapy can achieve some HPA-axis normalization.

Norepinephrine system. The norepinephrine (NE) system is also an integral part of human stress response (Goddard et al., 2010; Nestler, Hyman, & Malenka, 2009). Specifically, NE is thought to play a modulatory role in stress response, which may amplify or suppress anxiety depending on regulatory mechanisms (see Goddard et al., 2010). Noradrenergic nuclei have projections throughout the central nervous system, which means that changes in NE functioning can influence a wide range of biological manifestations, including executive processes (decision-making, attention), stress response, arousal/sleep, memory, and fear-learning. NE input also has a direct regulating mechanism on CRF (part of the HPA, described above), and thus can influence HPA activity. NE can also modulate signals from other neurotransmitters, including serotonin, dopamine, glutamate, and GABA. Acute and chronic stress can both affect NE functioning, with notable NE dysregulation being associated with pathological anxiety and depression in humans. The etiology is believed to be cyclical, with chronic stress dysregulating NE and NE dysfunction causing pathological anxiety and/or depression. Though the mechanisms are not yet fully understood, heightened NE activity and decreased NE receptor reactivity are both associated with clinically anxious patients. This is one of the reasons SNRIs are used in anxiety, in fact, because of their activity on NE reuptake. Given all the above, it is important to attempt to regulate NE system functioning in the treatment of anxiety disorders. However, contrary to HPA regulation (with studies measuring cortisol) currently, I am unaware of any research that specifically investigates changes in the NE system as a response to psychotherapy alone.

NE regulation is achieved through a number of medications, including some of the older antidepressants (tricyclics and MAOIs) as well as newer medications classified as SNRIs. These medications include venlafaxine (Effexor), desvenlafaxine (Pristiq), and duloxetine (Cymbalta). These medications can also be quite useful for anxiety and/or depression, but are usually tried only after an SSRI has been unsuccessful and are typically not prescribed routinely in pre-adolescent children. NE modulation also occurs through stimulants used in ADHD, though stimulants are not prescribed specifically for anxiety and can often worsen anxiety through dopamine withdrawal effects. Strattera (atomoxetine) is an often-used non-stimulant medication for ADHD that is a selective norepinephrine reuptake inhibitor (NRI). It generally has weaker effects on inattentive symptoms of ADHD than stimulants, but can sometimes be trialed in patients who do not tolerate stimulants and/or in patients who have a kind of "depressive" form of ADHD called "sluggish cognitive tempo" (Barkley, 2014). Another similar drug to atomoxetine, Qelbree (viloxazine), has gained popularity in the USA recently for use in ADHD, but comparative trials of Qelbree to other drugs are only just emerging at this time. Wellbutrin (bupropion) is another drug that inhibits the reuptake of NE, but it only does so weakly. Wellbutrin also weakly inhibits dopamine reuptake and very weakly inhibits serotonin reuptake. Its main mechanism of action is presumed to be through NE and dopamine (DA) reuptake interference. There are mixed findings about the efficacy of Wellbutrin for anxiety and depression (Patel et al., 2016), but it is typically a third- or fourth-line agent, after limited effect from other drugs being observed.

Still, there is rather little known about the actual unique, clinical (non-pharmacological) targets of these drugs, at least with regard to how they treat anxiety differently than other existing medications, and especially within the framework that is relevant to FELT. That is, I'm not sure noradrenergic drugs suggest alternative therapeutic action in addition to fulfillment and sedation/de-arousal, as outlined here. Regulating NE is important, but the chemical actions of NE do not produce any new therapeutic psychobehavioral targets that have not been discussed elsewhere.

The important therapeutic lesson that our discussion of NE does teach us is that nothing in the human mind and body exists in a vacuum. Every hormone and chemical interacts with something else, somewhere in the mind. The same can be said of psychobehavioral techniques. No one thing we do as therapists will sufficiently drive a child toward full healing. Instead, real healing is an integrative process, focused on many different areas of human functioning.

Behavioral and psychotherapeutic means to match biological needs

Throughout the preceding discussion on pharmacology and neurobiology of anxiety, some suggestions arose about how psychotherapists can think about the therapeutic targets of anxiety. In this section, I focus more closely on psychotherapeutic techniques which hone toward those same targets.

Fulfillment

The concept of fulfillment is perhaps too broad to provide full coverage here, but in FELT, fulfillment refers primarily to the fulfillment and healthy resolution of psychological needs described in detail in Chapter 4. By focusing on identifying where in their lives children are seeking fulfillment, but coming up "short," therapists can identify specific therapeutic targets to integrate into their directive Play Therapy. Using the metaphor provided by SSRIs – that if a person is given the opportunity to better use the serotonin they have, then they don't need more; they just need to be given a chance to actually receive what's already theirs to begin with – clinicians can practice more fluidly within the "amplifiers" and "suppressors" model of FELT outlined in Chapter 6. A major focus of FELT is to work to minimize amplifiers and maximize suppressors of the genetic risk for anxiety. In other words, we are helping to create an environment and internal psychology where children can fulfill a natural progression toward healthy resilience. This mentality can sometimes be "lost" in the field of clinical psychology, where often emphasis is placed on symptom reduction and treating clinical syndromes. Yes, FELT is being used to treat children with diagnosed anxiety disorders, so we are treating a clinical syndrome. However, in FELT, treatment is not "complete" simply when clinically significant symptoms are gone. **Rather, treatment is complete when a child reliably demonstrates an ability to fulfill within normal limits the psychological needs relevant to their development.**

Sedation/de-arousal

Anxiety can be a quite stressful physiological state. In extreme levels, it feels downright terrible. So, another major focus of anxiety management is learning how to make anxiety feel less terrible. For this reason, all existing evidence-based psychotherapies for anxiety and depression include some form of relaxation and mindfulness/meditation training. Examples of such techniques include relaxation training (Manzoni et al., 2008), interoceptive exposure (Boswell et al., 2013), and biofeedback (Knox et al., 2011). Each of these techniques has demonstrated long-term efficacy in regulating biological dysfunction associated with anxiety, with very few adverse side effects. The sedative effects of these exercises are a key clinical target in managing clinical anxiety in children. However, as any parent will tell you, most children resist "sedation" at least to some extent, and if given a choice between performing a quiet, relaxing activity, especially those involved in traditional meditation and muscle relaxation, versus an active one, most children express a preference for the active option. Thus, therapists often must adapt relaxation techniques to fit childhood preferences for "games" and "activity." These relaxation skills still have an anxiolytic effect in children even if they are not quiet or physiologically sedating/calming. What matters more is that children learn to use these techniques to reliably calm anxious states. Thus, they are focused on being psychologically sedating, even if physically children are still being quite active while using them.

So, when performing mindfulness/meditation with children, it is not always necessary to have them sit down in a chair, stay still, and meditate. Children can benefit from mindfulness practice through collaborative, imaginary storytelling, and children can even "act out" these stories in fun ways, while still practicing mindful attitudes. Similarly, progressive muscle relaxation (PMR) need not be the scripted "body scan" exercise that is often used in adults. Instead, PMR can include interactive games or exercise routines that involve PMR, or can be accomplished through traditional childhood games like "Simon Says." Likewise, biofeedback training does not have to be a "high-tech" option with electrodermal activity sensors and interactive computer games. Biofeedback can be accomplished simply by teaching children to attend to their heartbeat (perhaps through a stethoscope, feeling their pulse, or through a low-cost pulse oximeter) and then engaging in different activities to manipulate the heartbeat (i.e., exercise to speed up heart rate, relaxation to slow it down). Each of these activities is used in FELT and described further in Chapter 8, which outlines the actual FELT session content. Clinicians are encouraged to use these techniques to address biological dysfunction in all anxious children.

Chronic stress/anxiety also causes chronic HPA overactivity. Therapists can address HPA overactivity through a combination of teaching patients to use specific skills to minimize effects of stress and through environmental intervention to reduce or eliminate unnecessary or excessive environmental stressors. Methods for addressing HPA activity in individual children are similar to those described above in reviewing activities to mimic the sedative effects of drugs. However, one key difference is that HPA activity is managed through long-term and regular practice of these skills, *even when they are not necessarily needed to manage acute anxiety.* HPA activity, then, is regulated through daily skills practice and children are encouraged to use the skills even when they are not particularly anxious, as a way to help drive down the body's overall sensitivity when stressors do arise. Clinically anxious children are taught in developmentally appropriate terms about how their bodies have learned to overreact when stressors occur and that they can regain control over these reactions by training their body appropriately, similar to how athletes use exercise to prepare for sporting competitions.

Furthermore, childhood stress management is not only managed through relaxation and mindfulness training. In fact, more often than not, kids just want to have fun. So, finding ways to support children in having regular fun is also key to stress management. Kids should be encouraged to play, in every sense of the definition offered in Chapter 1. They need opportunities to be carefree and unfiltered, without negative affect getting in the way. They shouldn't always be completely free of negative affect, but they do benefit greatly from having room to de-stress through play. Such play, if balanced with other healthy exposures, will also balance and normalize HPA activity.

Attention to environmental stressors is also paramount in the management of HPA overactivity. It is not sufficient to simply teach children how to handle stress when it happens, though this is certainly important. It is also essential to normalize stressful exposures in children, as outlined in Chapter 6 (see "Environmental/cultural/learned factors"). Environmental stress should not be eliminated completely – this would be counterproductive and would more likely increase susceptibility to later anxiety than improve it. At the same time, major stressors should be addressed, and children are unlikely to benefit fully from psychotherapy if their lives are otherwise complicated by ongoing traumatic stressors.

Behavioral improvement of serotonin function

And another lesson from the efficacy of SSRIs, generalized negative affect seems at least partially driven by suboptimal serotonin activity, and boosting serotonin activity may contribute to positive therapeutic gains. Some research supports that behavioral and cognitive measures can alter serotonin metabolism in therapeutic ways. Perreau-Linck et al. (2007) found that self-reported happiness and sadness following specific mood-induction procedures correlated with serotonin synthesis in the brain (specifically, in the right cingulate cortex). This study showed clearly that mood/thought influences serotonin, just as serotonin influences mood/thought. In other words, serotonin use can be improved through psychological techniques, not just through medication. Similarly, exposure to bright light has been shown to increase serotonin as well, and these findings are fairly robust (Young, 2007).

A third strategy for increasing brain serotonin may be through exercise. Exercise has a well-established scientific link with boosted mood and decreased anxiety, and some emerging studies, particularly in animal studies, have shown increased serotonin levels following exercise (Young, 2007). A fourth serotonin management strategy can include diet. Specifically, scientists have investigated tryptophan consumption and its influence on serotonin. Serotonin is made from tryptophan in the body, and so tryptophan is a necessary precursor for serotonin synthesis. Consumption of purified tryptophan increases serotonin levels in the body, but eating foods that contain tryptophan does not (Wurtman, Hefti, & Melamed, 1980). The same is true of foods that contain serotonin (for example, bananas); these foods do not cross the blood–brain barrier and thus do not increase brain serotonin (Young, 2007). So, it is unlikely that consuming foods high in tryptophan is going to cause demonstrable increases in brain-available serotonin. However, having a full belly and satisfying nutritional needs certainly does have a beneficial effect on mood and overall mental health. So, even if direct effects cannot be achieved by eating serotonin or its precursors, indirect serotonin increases can certainly occur by following a nutritional, well-balanced diet.

So, four strategies emerge from this research review which can enhance natural serotonin levels and boost mental health: 1) a purposeful mental focus on positive, mood-boosting subjects; 2) intentional exposure to natural bright light (preferably >1000 lux); 3) regular exercise; and 4) a nutritionally complete, healthy, fulfilling diet.

Conclusion: key points from Part I of this book

In the next section of this book (Part II) we will move into describing the actual FELT session content, session-by-session. First though, it is important to review the key points outlined throughout Part I, to help condense these points into a more manageable format for recall. Returning to the FELT fidelity checklist first shown in Chapter 2 helps capture these key points. As a reminder, this checklist was used by FELT supervisors in early development studies to rate treatment fidelity among FELT providers. The entirety of Part I of this book was dedicated to giving therapists an in-depth understanding of what these components mean.

1 The therapy is play-based.
2 The play is characterized by metaphor and symbolism.
3 The therapist demonstrates clear evidence they have analyzed the child's play for themes.
4 The therapist uses themes to inform play-based responses.
5 The therapist is attuned to the child.
6 The therapist displays concern for the child.
7 The therapist intervenes therapeutically when opportunities arise.
8 The therapist is responsive to the child's direction.
9 The therapist is responsive to the child's needs.
10 The therapist is cautious about their interpretations and interventions.
11 The therapist uses clinically relevant material from the child's life narrative to understand and direct the symbolism in the play.

Of these 11 key points, the one that perhaps needs further commentary here is the eleventh one, which pertains to the child's "life narrative." In this case, what I really mean by "life narrative" is their individualized case conceptualization, as outlined in Chapters 6 and 7. In FELT development studies, FELT trainers/supervisors met with study therapists regularly to help promote fidelity and prepare for sessions. Study therapists were expected after session four to have a (mentally) prepared case conceptualization for each client to discuss in detail. Though I do not expect practicing clinicians to follow these study procedures exactly, I do think the timing of case conceptualizations is informative. It seems to take around four sessions for therapists to form a strong working conceptualization to be used in the latter two-thirds of therapy. Throughout the first month of therapy, in addition to providing therapy, therapists are also gathering data to inform a working model of the child's world as outlined in Figure 6.1.

Once they have those data in hand, therapists can now better work to understand and direct any symbolism that arises in the play. Specifically, they can more fluidly predict what unmet needs are being expressed in the play, and they can intervene through play to resolve those needs in a healthy manner. Outside of play, they can also look to environmental and biological determinants that also need intervention.

These 11 characteristics of FELT infiltrate every technique we will now see in Part II.

Notes

1 Of course, most medications will hit those neurochemical targets much more powerfully than any behavioral method can achieve, and many children do benefit from using medication to supplement and/or facilitate gains.
2 Though MAOIs are still a viable treatment for depression, they are not selective about what neurotransmitters they affect. MAO will trash all of the monoamines, including serotonin, norepinephrine, and dopamine, so blocking MAO means an increase in all these neurotransmitters, which isn't usually ideal. MAOIs have far more side effects and drug–drug/drug–food interactions than newer antidepressants.
3 The need for fulfillment can derive from several of the basic needs covered in Chapter 4. For example, if fulfillment represents a feeling of empowerment, independence, freedom, or authority, it comes from *exousia* and *dunamis* needs. If fulfillment is relationship based, it can represent a need for love, need for Objects, or popularity needs, depending on the nature of the relationship. Fulfillment should not be understood here as an additional basic human need, but rather a journey toward other basic needs.
4 Obviously, the usage of ECT for depression pertains to adults. ECT should never be used or recommended for children.

REFERENCES

Barkley, R. A. (2014). Sluggish cognitive tempo (concentration deficit disorder?): current status, future directions, and a plea to change the name. *Journal of Abnormal Child Psychology*, 42(1), 117–125.

Boswell, J. F., Farchione, T. J., Sauer-Zavala, S., Murray, H. W., Fortune, M. R., & Barlow, D. H. (2013). Anxiety sensitivity and interoceptive exposure: a transdiagnostic construct and change strategy. *Behavior Therapy*, 44(3), 417–431.

Castro-Vale, I., & Carvalho, D. (2020). The pathways between cortisol-related regulation genes and PTSD psychotherapy. *Healthcare*, 8(4), 376.

Gengo, F. M., Dabronzo, J., Yurchak, A., Love, S., & Miller, J. K. (1987). The relative antihistaminic and psychomotor effects of hydroxyzine and cetirizine. *Clinical Pharmacology and Therapeutics*, 42(3), 265–272.

Goddard, A. W., Ball, S. G., Martinez, J., Robinson, M. J., Yang, C. R., Russell, J. M., & Shekhar, A. (2010). Current perspectives of the roles of the central norepinephrine system in anxiety and depression. *Depression and Anxiety*, 27(4), 339–350.

Knox, M., Lentini, J., Cummings, T. S., McGrady, A., Whearty, K., & Sancrant, L. (2011). Game-based biofeedback for paediatric anxiety and depression. *Mental Health in Family Medicine*, 8(3), 195–203.

Laurent, H. K., Gilliam, K. S., Wright, D. B., & Fisher, P. A. (2015). Child anxiety symptoms related to longitudinal cortisol trajectories and acute stress responses: evidence of developmental stress sensitization. *Journal of Abnormal Psychology*, 124(1), 68–79.

Manzoni, G. M., Pagnini, F., Castelnuovo, G., & Molinari, E. (2008). Relaxation training for anxiety: a ten-years systematic review with meta-analysis. *BMC Psychiatry*, 8, 41.

Nestler, E. J., Hyman, S. E., & Malenka, R. C. (2009). *Molecular Neuropharmacology: A Foundation for Clinical Neuroscience*. New York: McGraw-Hill.

Parker, A. J., Hamlin, G. P., Coleman, C. J., & Fitzpatrick, L. A. (2003). Dehydration in stressed ruminants may be the result of a cortisol-induced diuresis. *Journal of Animal Science*, 81(2), 512–519.

Patel, K., Allen, S., Haque, M. N., Angelescu, I., Baumeister, D., & Tracy, D. K. (2016). Bupropion: a systematic review and meta-analysis of effectiveness as an antidepressant. *Therapeutic Advances in Psychopharmacology*, 6(2), 99–144.

Perreau-Linck, E., Beauregard, M., Gravel, P., Paquette, V., Soucy, J. P., Diksic, M., & Benkelfat, C. (2007). In vivo measurements of brain trapping of ^{11}C-labelled α-methyl-L-tryptophan during acute changes in mood states. *Journal of Psychiatry and Neuroscience*, 32(6), 430–434.

Steadman, J. (2016). Evidence-based practice in play-analysis: interpreting and using the play of anxious children. *British Journal of Play Therapy*, 12, 52–75.

Wurtman, R. J., Hefti, F., & Melamed, E. (1980). Precursor control of neurotransmitter synthesis. *Pharmacology Review*, 32(4), 315–335.

Young, S. N. (2007). How to increase serotonin in the human brain without drugs. *Journal of Psychiatry and Neuroscience*, 32(6), 394–399.

Part II

Session guides and story stem creation

Chapter 8

The FELT treatment outlined by session

Armed with the theories and evidence base outlined thus far, it is now time to enter into the actual session content of FELT. As noted numerous times so far in this book, FELT is a comprehensive *approach* to psychotherapy with children, and thus includes far more techniques and theory than are contained in the following session-by-session outlines. Therefore, it is important for clinicians as they move through these FELT sessions to retain in mind the other lessons outlined so far that are key to FELT – that is, evidence-based play analysis, Object-relations and Self theories, therapeutic mechanisms of change, and the FELT etiological model. These ideas will be referenced throughout the sessions outlined in this chapter.

Before starting FELT – materials needed

Each FELT session was designed to fit within the standard 45-minute "therapy hour." The procedures have been tested with many kids and session content was tweaked in early trials to ensure goals could be reached with the majority of kids within the allotted time. Furthermore, in studies, FELT was administered weekly, in general, with allowances for delaying a session as needed to accommodate client and therapist schedules (e.g., needing to cancel occasionally due to illness, vacation, etc.). Ideally then, therapists implementing FELT should plan to execute around twelve 45- to 50-minute sessions, scheduled on a weekly basis.

Therapists will also need some essential play-supplies (toys) to accomplish session goals. A list of essential supplies is included below. Therapists may use any variation of toy/supply as needed to fit the needs listed below. In FELT studies, different sites used different toys, and most play therapists will likely already have most of these supplies on hand in their existing collection.

Guidelines for all sessions

The session-by-session guides below will advise therapists about a typical progression of play stems used to organize FELT and to accomplish specific therapeutic goals. Still, therapists should recall from Part I of this book that FELT is at its core a child-responsive intervention, and so therapists are

DOI: 10.4324/9781032693187-10

Table 8.1 List of items/toys needed for FELT

Category	Item	Comment
People toys	Multiple adults, male and female[1] Multiple children, male and female Doctor(s) Police Robbers	See footnote 1 for comment about genders. Archetypal toys – that is, those that are meant to represent specific professions or characteristics (doctor, police, robbers) – do not always have to obviously match their archetype. Any toy can become a "doctor" if we just assign the title to the toy. Still, it can be helpful to have some toys that obviously "pull" for certain traits. This creates a structure for children that is useful in FELT and helps to keep story stems more predictable and controlled. The toys named here – doctor, police, robbers – are the three archetypes that fill necessary roles in FELT story stems. But most play therapists should also have other archetypal toys too (e.g., heroes, villains, etc.).
Animal toys	Predator and prey toys (any combination, several of each) Adult and baby (animal families) Wild and domestic Common pets (dogs and cats, especially); will need at least three birds: two parrots and one toucan*	Two parrots and one toucan are used in one story stem to mimic catastrophic thinking during an anxious episode. In the story, the toucan gets frightened because it has a "huge beak" while the parrots have a "normal beak." Thus, any set of three animals of similar species, where one has a distinct physical difference from the other two, can be used for this stem.
Buildings	Clinic House School Fences Cage	These buildings do not have to be clearly designed for each use (i.e., any building can serve as a make-shift clinic or school). Therapists on a tight budget can also create buildings/partitions from cardboard boxes if necessary. Fences and cage can be any kind of partition – in FELT stems these are commonly used as "containers"/barriers to provide safety for characters.

Category	Item	Comment
Plants	Trees Bushes Rocks	These are used to create settings/homes for animal toys, and, occasionally, as natural partitions/barriers (i.e., climbing a tree to escape a predator, hiding behind rocks).
Vehicles	Cars/transport large enough for people toys – two types are advised	In one story stem, a mobile vet clinic is created in which a vet drives out to the jungle to help some birds, thus, a safari-like jeep can help with the "realism" of this stem, but any car will do.
Furniture/ Tools	Tables Chairs Desks Computer Kitchen tools (plates, cups, utensils) School-related supplies (books, pencils/pens, laboratory equipment) Medical supplies (cast, scalpel, shots, ultrasound machine) Nurturing supplies (food, bottles, drinks) Valuables (money, jewels, artifacts) Weapons (knives, guns, clubs)	Ideally, these items are sized to fit the available people toys.
Other	Real, working stethoscope (two of them) Blue cloth, paper, or other material (used to represent a body of water) Large cardboard box Large stackable blocks Sticky notes	Stethoscopes should function properly, but need not be high quality. They will be used to detect a heartbeat at the left-lower sternal border (LLSB) to measure heart rate in beats per minute. They do not need to be capable of detecting murmurs or other cardiac abnormalities. Large cardboard box is typically around three to four feet tall when flattened. Large stackable blocks should be large enough to stack four to five of them to reach the top of the large cardboard box (see session 6 for more details).

encouraged every session to put the child's responsiveness and needs ahead of any particular session format or play stem. In other words, the general goals of each session and the child's individual needs, preferences, and play skill take precedence over the need to perfectly execute story stems as written here.

Just because a certain story stem is included in a session does not mean that a therapist cannot adapt the stem to better fit an individual child.

Also, in all sessions, a certain amount of free play and exploration by the child is permissible. Especially in early sessions, it is important to draw a balance between introducing FELT as a structured play format while also leaving room for the child to play their own ideas, while still remaining faithful to key treatment values and specific session goals. For example, it is expectable that a child may initiate some fantasy play that keys into an anxious issue for the child, even before the therapist intended to open that issue in a session. If this occurs, therapists can respond accordingly and follow the child's lead in helping with that issue. It is important not to discourage therapeutic play just because it happens "too early" in therapy. At the same time, FELT skills are designed to be taught/learned in a stepwise basis, building upon each other over time to maximize the efficacy of therapy. So, as children direct their own ideas into play, it is still important for therapists to maintain focus on the stepwise fashion of therapeutic goals.

Still, because children are prone toward spontaneous (and potentially "off-topic") play, therapists are advised to use FELT session goals and story stems to control the specific toys available to a child during session. Rather than making all toys in the playroom available for the child to use as desired, it often works better to select the toys necessary for the session and to limit the child to using those. By limiting toy selection, therapists maintain better control over the direction of the session and also help reduce natural exploratory play that happens when children are exposed to new toys. Nevertheless, children should still be allowed agency to choose preferred toys from the available selection. If a story stem calls for a child, a dog, and two parents, then the child is instructed to choose from all the available toys (say, 50 or so options of "people" toys) the specific toys they want to represent each role. Occasionally, therapists may learn through trials that certain children struggle to make such choices if they are given too many options or that they take too long to choose their toys. In these cases, the therapist can increase efficiency by reducing the number of options available or by simply choosing the specific toys themselves.

In tracking play themes, beginning therapists may benefit from making brief written notes during sessions about what themes were noted. If written notes are made during session, it is highly advised that therapists do so in as unobtrusive a manner as possible, and without interrupting the flow of a play narrative. Often, beginning therapists learning FELT have used session cue cards containing an outline of key session goals and activities. These cue cards are included in this manual. Beginning therapists may also benefit from a themes cue card, reminding them of the core themes and on which they may choose to mark simple tallies of themes as they arise. However, again, therapists should work to have enough facility with session materials and basic thematic analysis that they can execute sessions without relying too frequently on notes. Again, the key goal is to allow the child to experience a narrative flow in play, and that the therapist is engaged and collaborating with them in the play. In other words, if a therapist finds themselves acting exclusively as an observer of the child's play, but not a participant, then questions should arise about what can be done differently to engage and interact more regularly with the child and their play. In FELT, it is essential for the therapist to be active in play.

Session descriptions in this chapter have been written from the basis that toys are used to create scenes and therapeutic narratives. However, some children may express dislike of the particular toys available and may instead prefer alternative methods of play. In such cases, therapists are encouraged to adapt play materials to fit a child's particular interests and "play language." For example, some children may gravitate toward puppet play, rather than figure-based play. Others may prefer other expressive artistic endeavors, such as theater, visual arts, or music. Any form of expressive therapy can work in FELT, as long as therapists find a way to stick to the narrative, story-based form of each intervention. Children who prefer puppets or theater can simply enact the story stems through role-play with the therapist. Children who prefer visual arts may choose to draw story stems and then tell stories about the artwork. These adaptations have all been used in FELT clinical trials as needed and have been shown to be equally effective adaptations of the FELT model. Musical adaptations, on the other hand, have not been investigated in research at this time. In fact, musical adaptations may not be realistically possible in FELT for most children, as the compositional skill necessary to follow the narrative nature of FELT through music is usually not yet developed in young and elementary-age children. Theoretically, musical narratives could be applied according to the FELT structure, but this application would need much more research before it could be implemented on a regular basis. Still, there are many expressive therapies aside from the figure-based play described in FELT sessions below, and so therapists should not feel they must always adhere to the exact toys and figures described, as long as core session goals are still met, and as long as the structure of the expressive play leaves room for story stems and analyses of how these stems are then resolved.

Session 1

Purpose

To get to know one another. To explain and model basic information about the treatment. To begin to gather information about situations that make the child anxious and the child's reactions to signs of anxiety.

Goals

1 Build rapport
2 Orient child to the program
3 Gather information about child's preferences and style of play and communication

Methods

Begin by introducing yourself in a calm, child-responsive manner. Children with anxiety disorders can be avoidant, fearful, or wary, and may not be comfortable with direct questions asked too quickly in the course of therapy. As therapist, you should be attentive to the child's cues and should approach in a manner that is respectful of those cues. Once a basic introduction is made, ample time should be devoted to establishing a trusting relationship in which the child can begin to feel safe when in your presence as the therapist. The activities in this session are designed to allow a friendly, playful exchange to begin.

At some point during the first session, you may verbally orient the child to the structure of the FELT. When the child seems ready, you should communicate three "rules" about the play therapy, in order of importance:

1 Everyone must always be safe, all the time.
2 The therapist and the child both get to decide what feels safe and what does not.
3 (Usually communicated as the therapist begins to prepare the first story stem) "When we play together here, most of the time we will play stories together. I'll start the stories, and then we'll finish them together. You can play anything you want, as long as you use the toys I give you. We will always try to finish a story before you leave, too."

There are several purposes for establishing these three rules. First, it is made clear that the therapist is concerned with helping the child feel safe. This "rule" creates a boundary for what play happens in therapy, but it also communicates concern and care toward the child, a core feature of the ACER characteristics outlined in Chapter 5. Second, the therapist communicates that the child's point of view matters, and that the therapist will respect the child's fears when appropriate. Again, on the surface, this rule establishes that neither therapist nor child will violate each other's boundaries and that the therapist will not ask the child to do anything that is not safe. The second rule is also a subtle message that collaborative decisions are a hallmark of therapy. Although as adults, therapists do retain some authority over the session content, the child will also be offered a say in what happens in sessions. Third, the general structure of the play intervention is described. This helps establish up front that play will follow a specific structure and will help reduce later deviations from the story-stem structure. It is essential to establish the story-stem structure from the first session; otherwise, children may get the wrong idea about what is supposed to happen in Play Therapy and may begin to introduce too much unstructured play that can render the remaining FELT structure untenable.

Activity 1: Getting to know each other

There are many ways to build rapport in a first session, and many therapists may have their own preferred ways to do so. The following activity is recommended because it helps accomplish all three of the core goals of this session (building rapport, orienting child to the program, and gathering information about preferred styles of play and general play skill). It also allows the child to engage in exploratory play with most, if not all, of the figures that will be used throughout FELT. By allowing the child to conduct a full "scan" of exploratory play in session 1, it reduces later exploratory play and thus allows later sessions to flow more efficiently.

To begin the session, allow the child to sort through all the toys that may be used throughout FELT. The child is told that they are going to play a game where "I (the therapist) get to learn about you." Instruct the child to, "Choose some toys from the box [or table, or wherever you keep the toys] that will tell me about you." While the child is searching, consider toys to choose to represent yourself, but do not make your choice until the child has settled upon their own choice(s). You should not offer interpretive comments while the child is choosing (wait until after all choices are made for this), but you should be responsive to any questions or comments the child makes themself. The child may play with or explore any of the toys briefly, but if this detracts too much from the task, a gentle reminder may be applied such as, "Is that the one you wanted to choose to be you?" Once the child has chosen, make benign inquisitions about the toy, using your own toy to speak to the child's toy (except for the first question, see below). The following are some potential questions/invitations to ask. You may ask these questions even if you have already done so as therapist in a previous session (i.e., during intake). The purpose here is to establish that you and the child will use the toys to talk to each other and to establish comfort with the playful nature of FELT.

1   As therapist (not as toy you chose) open with, "Tell me about this toy."
    (If necessary, add, "...and how it is like you.")
2   (Using toy) What's your middle name?
3   How old are you?
4   How many brothers and sisters do you have?
5   What's your favorite TV show?
6   Do you have any favorite heroes (or superheroes)?
7   And so on.

The child may ask you similar questions about your own toy. Be prepared to provide answers as appropriate. Therapists usually work to choose toys for themselves (as therapists) that also reflect their role in the therapeutic relationship. For example, therapists may choose a "doctor" toy to help delineate their role as a doctor or they may choose a tree and say something like, "I chose a tree for myself because trees are safe little homes for animals, a place where animals can relax and just be themselves, and that reminds me of my job, because my job is to help kids feel safe, relax, and just be themselves." Your selection and description of your own Self-toys is a vital component of outlining for children the purpose of sessions and of describing who you are and what your job is.

Also, *make a (mental) note of the toy(s) chosen by the child as the Self.* FELT studies have shown that children will often return to these toys when selecting toys that represent the Self in later narratives, even when not instructed to choose a "Self-toy," and so it is important for therapists to recall which toys the child identifies most closely with, and what features of the child's Self-identity are activated by various toys. The child may also ask if they can pick toys to represent his/her family members. The child may be allowed to do so if they ask but are not required to.

One final consideration for this activity is whether certain toys should be excluded from the procedure. I advocate strongly for having a wide range of toys for this activity, including both animal and people toys. In some forms of Play Therapy, it is important to have "neutral" toys, on which the child may project aspects of the Self, which aids in play analysis. In these forms of Play Therapy, there is a need to allow a "purer" analysis of play content, so analysis is not encumbered by the inherent characteristics of certain toys. For example, a "Superman" toy will almost always be used as a powerful, benevolent superhero and thus is a less flexible toy and not as much of a "blank canvas." At the same time, a Superman toy who is depicted as a bad guy or as weak requires the child to negate the archetypal components that make Superman who he is. So, to "erase" the core components of Superman's identity can be quite meaningful in play analysis, potentially suggesting that the child may have their own questions about the reliability of identity and the consistency of the Self. For these reasons, FELT encourages the usage of both neutral AND archetypal toys throughout and especially in this first activity. Having archetypal toys – those that overtly call for certain characteristics – is quite useful in this introductory activity. It creates a structure to allow children to identify role models in their selection of Self-representative toys, and it opens new possibilities for investigating abstract characteristics in young children who struggle with abstraction. If offered only neutral toys, young children will tend to identify those that share physical characteristics – "I chose this one because it has a pink shirt, and I'm wearing a pink shirt today." However, if archetypal toys are available, the archetypal characteristics of these toys often elicit more abstract relating – "I chose this policeman because I want to be a policeman when I'm older," and they allow the therapist more "material" to which to react – "Oh, you want to be a policeman? What do you like about policemen?" So, in FELT, and in this activity in particular, therapists should strive to make available a combination of both "neutral" and "archetypal" toys to the child.

It is also important in this activity to recall that this session is likely to be children's first exposure to all the toys in your collection. Consequently, children will be inclined to explore the toys in detail. It is not uncommon for this activity alone to take as much as 15–20 minutes of therapy time, due to the child wanting to inventory and explore your toy collection. Thus, to help reduce distractions of exploratory play, therapists should consider excluding toys that may warrant an extended exploration. Action figures that have moving components, vehicles that transform into robots, and toys that make noise should probably be excluded from this procedure. They can be saved for later sessions when they can be explored in isolation, away from the cumulative exploration of all the other toys.

Activity 2: Introduction to therapy

This activity flows somewhat naturally from activity 1. Now is the time to begin to introduce story stems, as they will be used throughout FELT. The first story stem is meant primarily to orient the child to the program. You will want to make the following points during this activity:

1   The program is a joint effort between the therapist and child.
2   There are reasons the child is coming to see the therapist, which may be described with some variation of any of the following:

   a   "Some kids need help with _____, and I am here to try to help them..."
   b   "All kids worry about something. My job is to help them figure out what they worry about and try to help them not worry so much."

3   Begin to discuss goals for treatment, including being able to identify anxious feelings and making sense of how those feelings fit into the child's life.
4   Stress that the child's point of view is very important.

To make these points, the following story stem was designed.
Toys needed: child's Self-toy, therapist's Self-toy, clinic, other environment-specific toys.

Introduction: [As you collect relevant toys] "When you come here to see me, we're going to do something special. Often when you come here, I'm going to take certain toys from this box, and I'm going to make up a story for you to finish for me. I'll start the story, and then it will be your turn to tell me how it ends. We'll play with the toys together until we both feel like the story is finished. Let's do the first one now so you can get an idea of what it's like."

Story: The point of this story stem is to attempt to recreate the child's experience of entering the current treatment environment. Thus, extra toys may be chosen as necessary to help simulate any child-specific or environment-specific factors (e. g., if the child was seated with the mother before coming into therapy, you may ask the child to help you choose a "mommy toy" to be the mother in this story). The first part of the story stem will be to set up the toys to reflect how you met the child (that day), how you retrieved them from the waiting room, and how you brought them back to the therapy room. Thus, the first part of the story stem will vary depending on the environment, how the child reacted, and so on. You will narrate the story as you remember it, using the relevant toys to enact the scene. The child may change features to match their own perspective, and this should be allowed and responded to accordingly, even if they do not match your memory of the scene. After the characters move inside the clinic, the following story stem should be played:

[Key: T = therapist's Self-toy; C = child's Self-toy]

T: "Hello [name]. How are you today?"
C: "I'm okay, but I'm not sure why I'm here."
T: "You're not? Well, do you know what I do?"
C: "No."
T: "A lot of kids worry about things. My job is to help them figure out…" [see points and variations above]. "Why don't you tell me about what you'd like to do in here…" [Hand over control to child by saying] "Now you finish this story."

As the child finishes, you should be responsive and interact as necessary, helping to make the points listed previously. Use the play to communicate treatment goals and how story stems will be used to address those goals.

Activity 3: A happy time

Builds rapport. Introduces task of playing about feelings, but uses a "safe" feeling. This activity does not use a story stem, but follows a more open-ended, child-directed play format.

Toys needed: child chooses.

Introduction: "Let's play about a happy time. Let's choose some toys to play a happy time. What kind of happy time do you want to play?"

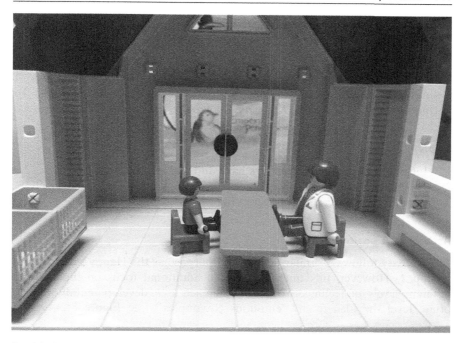

Fig. 8.1 A basic set-up of the child–therapist play interview. Photo by author.

Child may inquire if the happy time has to be personal. This activity does not require the happy time to be about the child. This is simply any happy time.

Work with and follow the child to create a happy scene. Have the child narrate you through what happens, as the child simultaneously enacts the narration. The scene may be very detailed or may be quite basic. Make a mental note of how skilled the child appears to be at engaging in fantasy play. "Good" players are expected to benefit more from Play Therapy than "poor" players. If the child is a "poor" player, you, as therapist, may need to take a more directive lead throughout FELT to engage the child in play and teach the child important play skills. Thus, the information you obtain about the quality of the child's fantasy will serve to inform your therapeutic process later.

In reacting to the content of the Happy time stem, it can be helpful as a precedent, in preparation for session 2, to comment and/or ask some basic questions about what "happy" feels like and/or looks like. So, when the child enacts happy characters, you may take control of a character and provide commentary such as, "This is so fun! I feel so happy! I am going to smile all day long, and I feel like I am just floating!" Similarly, you may ask the child to describe themselves what happy is like. If they struggle with this, it is not essential to push the point today, and you may instead focus on modeling happy through your own commentary as exemplified above.

Session 2 – "Feelings are important"

Purpose

To review goals of treatment. To help the child identify different types of feelings and to distinguish anxious, worried feelings from other kinds. To normalize feelings of fear and anxiety. To explore the child's sense of anxiety.

Goals

1   Introduce that different feelings have different expressions
2   Normalize fears and anxiety
3   Begin to construct anxiety hierarchy

Activity 1: A positive feeling

This activity follows a similar format and purpose as the Happy time story in session 1. However, this time, there is an additional focus on highlighting different levels of feelings. You may reference at a developmentally appropriate level the idea of an "emotions circumplex" (see Figure 8.2), which

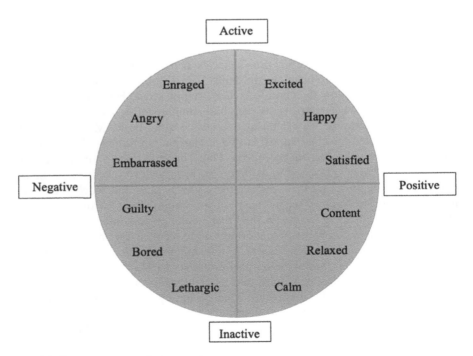

Fig. 8.2 Emotions circumplex: example

highlights that feelings can vary on two dimensions, valence (positive vs. negative) and intensity/arousal-level (active vs. inactive). For this activity, we focus on different levels of positive feelings. In other session 2 activities, we introduce a circumplex of negative feelings.

Introduction: "Remember last session when we ended by playing about a happy time. Today, we are going to do something similar, but this time, we will play about other kinds of feelings. Let's start with a good feeling. What are some different kinds of good feelings?"

For some children, it may be helpful to provide a list of potential feelings from which the child can choose. During the treatment development studies, the following feelings were most frequently used, but other positive feelings may be chosen by the child if desired.

1   Excited
2   Loved
3   Playful
4   Surprised

Once they've chosen a feeling, help them create a story around this feeling. It is often useful to help kids "plan" the story before they grab toys and start. This planning gives them structure and helps decrease chances the child will get "sidetracked" and start playing something else. So, talk to them about a time they've felt the feeling they chose, and then, once they've described the memory, help recreate that memory through play.

Throughout the scene, be sure to have the child label how she knows she feels the chosen emotion. You may ask, for example, "What does excited feel like?" or, "What happens inside [the character's] body when he/she is excited?" You may also reference the Happy time story from session 1 and set a comparison between the "happy" in session 1 and the positive feeling in session 2. You can use any child-appropriate rating scale for this – a 0–10 number system, a stack of blocks – anything that can represent scale for the child to compare the intensity of their session 1 happy and this session 2 positive feeling. This will help the child get used to a rudimentary "rating system" for various intensities of emotion. You should allot approximately 15–20 minutes for this activity, so as to leave time for activities 2 and 3.

Activity 2: Worry time

Introduction: "We just played about times when kids are [happy, excited, loved, playful, etc.]. But sometimes kids get scared feelings too. Sometimes they worry about things. All kids do it. I'm going to start a story about a time when a kid might be worried, and I want you to help me finish it."

Toys needed: child, parents, dog, table, container (for juice).

Story stem (Spilled juice): this stem is very similar to one used in the MacArthur Story Stem Battery (MSSB), referenced in Chapter 2. In order to make the best use of the MSSB evidence base, the spilled juice stem was included in FELT as a low-level trigger of a potentially anxiety-provoking situation, to help introduce topics of anxiety while exploring a child's reactions early in the course of intervention.

To set up the Spilled juice stem, you should ask the child to choose the necessary toys outlined above. Once choices are made, you then set up a room with a child, dog, table, and container (of juice) on the table. Next, you set up another room and place the parents inside, with commentary that they are "watching TV" in that room while the child plays with their dog in the other room. It is often useful to set things up in a house (e.g., a dollhouse), which can allow the child to be sent to their room or run away to their room if they choose to do so. If a house is not available, a third room can be set up to represent the child's bedroom.

After setup is complete, you introduce the story stem as follows, acting out the scene as you go. For simplicity, we will assume the child character in this example is a girl. "This little girl is playing with her dog, and they are having a great time. The dog is running around, jumps in the girl's lap, gives her kisses, and the girl is very happy playing with her dog. She gets thirsty and decides to go take a drink of grape juice. She goes to take a drink, and then she sets the cup back on the table, but, oops, she makes a mistake when she goes to put it back and the juice falls on the floor and spills all over the place. The parents heard the noise and come in to check what happened. They see the juice all over the floor. What happens next?"

Here, you allow the child to take over play as you follow along as needed. In my experience with FELT, most (>75%) children respond to this stem with very little to no anxiety. They either clean up the juice themselves or have the parents clean it up, and then the scene is over. In these cases, the entire story can last less than two minutes, and there is little material to which to react to explore anxiety as intended. Some children may respond with more overt anxiety, blaming the spill on the dog (in fact, this is the reason for including the dog in the stem, to allow this possibility), for example, or having the parents get angry and send the child to her room. In either case, there are five key points you want to try to elicit from the play or from the child:

1 What did the child think would happen?
2 What did she feel?
3 How did she know she felt that feeling?

    a May include an internalized "sense" of the feeling, somatic cues, behavioral manifestations, etc.

4 How did she act in response to how she felt?
5 How are the child's feelings in the spilled juice story different from those described in the "positive feelings" story?

Even when the child does not express clear anxiety through play (i.e., they clean up the mess without any incident), you can still return to the scene and elicit responses to these questions: "How did she feel right when her parents walked in?" "How did that feeling compare to how the other characters felt in your Happy stem earlier?"

If anxious themes arise, and the child does not herself do anything through the play to resolve those feelings of anxiety, the therapist should use suggestions in symbolic play to model how the child might address her anxiety. For example, consider the following scenario (again, this would be a rather extreme reaction to the Spilled juice stem, very rarely seen in FELT studies. It is used here for illustrative purposes only. If a child actually responds to the Spilled juice stem as is outlined in this fictional case, you should ask yourself as therapist why such an unusual response occurred and plan to respond accordingly either in this or in future sessions).

Example 1

> The child finishes the story as follows: "The girl blames the dog. Parents scold the girl. Girl insists the dog did it. Parents ground the girl for lying. Girl kicks the dog as she walks to her room."

Several themes are apparent in this scene. First, the girl shows anxiety, and copes by denying herself the experience of resolving that anxiety and instead projects blame elsewhere. Her parents are misattuned to the anxiety and fail to respond to the child's emotional needs by simply punishing the behavior without making an effort to communicate attunement, concern, and responsiveness. As a result, the girl becomes more distressed. Not knowing how to manage that distress, she kicks the dog in frustration and leaves the situation.

So, in summary, the therapist should note maladaptive themes of anxiety, subjugation/avoidance of the anxiety, punitiveness (the girls expects punishment, hence why she becomes anxious at all, and the parents execute it), lack of responsiveness, and, finally, surrender (that it won't get better, so just give up and leave). In FELT terms, these themes translate to negative initial and final content. There is resolution of content, but the resolution is clearly negative. There is a slight emotional shift from (implied) anxiety (trying to avoid punishment by lying) to frustrative anger (kicking the dog) and a major emotional shift from the joy of the story stem to the purely negative affect in the story resolution. Affect is rather incongruent, especially when considering the rarity of such an intense response to the Spilled juice stem. The child does not label any emotions in this scene, nor does she label any symptoms. Self-representations are ineffective and disorganized, while "Other" representations are that parents/authority figures are depicted as prone to punitiveness and short-temperedness.

Given these themes, the therapist should now strive to develop a play-based intervention that introduces alternatives to the child. In the current scenario, a primary source of the problem is the internal Object-relation between the child and parents, that the parents are misattuned and unresponsive to the child's needs, instead focused on the behavior (the fact she lied) and immediately scolding, rather than working through the fear. Inside this Object-relation, mistakes are not safe. If this problem is a recurring one in the child's life, the therapist should expect to work with the parents to instruct them how they may respond better. Accordingly, part of the intervention in the current play can model for the child what the therapist may do with the parents to teach them how they may help the child. The therapists works to correct this particular Object-relation by intervening with the Object.

So, the therapist may introduce another character in the play, preferably the "therapist-Self" toy, although others could be used. That character may come to speak to the parents about what happened, and may talk with them about the child's experience and teach them how to respond better.

THERAPIST: "I was watching everything and I wonder if maybe [name] spilled the juice on accident and then she got really worried that she was going to get in trouble. I don't think she knew that it was okay to be that worried."
PARENTS: "She was worried? Then why didn't she just tell us? Instead, she lied and then hurt the dog."
T: "Well, I wonder if maybe she just didn't really know. Do you think she was just thinking about the mess she made? Maybe she was so worried you'd be mad that she couldn't even figure out what to say? Maybe there is some way we can all help her figure it out? Why don't we try the scene again and see how we can help."

Then, the scene can be repeated, with the therapist guiding the parents and child toward a healthier resolution. Here is an example. Picking up at the end of the stem, when the parents come in, the therapist toy speaks first.

THERAPIST TOY: "Okay, here [name] has spilled her juice. She's probably thinking, 'Uh oh – I'm going to be in so much trouble.' She's scared, is that right?"

Looks to the child toy for a response. The child confirms. "Yes. I don't want to be in trouble." THERAPIST TOY: "Alright, mom and dad, let's try this. Let's see what happens if we don't get mad, but instead we check first to see how [blank] feels."

Switching to the parent toys, the therapist plays the parents. Since this is an early session, it's probably best for the therapist to direct the outcome by speaking for the parent toys here. If this scene or a similar one were played in later therapy, after some therapeutic gains were made, the therapist may choose to allow the child to speak for the parents, as a means to more directly explore, for themself, a healthier Object-relation. Still, because we are still early in treatment, the therapist in this example is intentionally directing a healthier Object-relation, to demonstrate for the child what is possible.

> Speaking as the parent toys: "Whoa. That was a scary sound. Are you okay?" [Here, you are modeling an acknowledgment of an internal state – being "scared."]
> Perhaps the child responds, "The juice got spilled!"
> "Oh. That's okay. Mistakes happen, and we can clean it up together. Let's get some towels." They then proceed to clean up together. "Do you feel okay now? You can keep playing with the dog if you want." The child takes over play briefly here and resumes playing with the dog, having a good time again.

In this re-play, the child is able to see an example of a healthier exchange between parents and child. In this case, parents are attuned and responsive. In terms of FELT themes, we also see a neutral initial response and a positive final resolution of content. We have labeled emotions, and we resolved those emotions too (the child resumes playing at the end, as if the spill never happened). We see a Self-representation that is more normative – kids make mistakes, and those mistakes are okay – and healthier other-representations – that caring adults will help you recover from your mistakes when needed. So, as therapist, we have taken all the notable problematic themes from the first play-through and we have corrected them succinctly.

Activity 3: Client-specific anxiety

If timing of the first two activities was performed appropriately, then you should have about 15 minutes remaining for this final story. For some children, 15 minutes is not enough to complete a full, self-driven story. Thus, it is important to carefully manage time in this final activity to maximize the chances you will be able to resolve the anxiety in this story before the end of the session.

Introduction: "We just played a scene that I made up where the child in the scene was worried. Now I wonder if maybe you want to try to make one up? You can use any of the toys to show me what 'scared' or 'worried' is like. What do you think?"

If the child agrees, proceed accordingly, helping to set up the scene as you did for the happy scene. As above, if maladaptive responses to anxiety become apparent through the play, respond accordingly. Consistent with overall session goals, you should focus attention not only to describing anxiety sufficiently; you should also help the child highlight similarities and differences to the other two story stems, again helping familiarize the child to the process of rating varying intensities of emotion. Example 2, below, shows a potential response and intervention by the therapist.

If the child is unable to create a spontaneous anxiety-focused story on their own, or they otherwise detract from the task, it could be a sign that the child is not yet ready to explore such an avenue into their negative emotional state (they could also just be having a form of "writer's block"). If this occurs, reassure the child that it is okay they couldn't come up with anything just yet, that maybe they can do one another time if they want, and to let you know if they change their mind. Then, offer a second scene of your own. You may use the one described in Example 2, or you may create one of your own. If you do create one of your own, you should avoid creating a scene that you might expect to relate too directly to an anxiety-provoking reality for the child, given it is still early in therapy and you have not been able to evaluate their readiness for such a stem.

Example 2

Toys used: alligator, snake, gorillas (adult and baby), tree, fence.

The child creates a scene where a baby gorilla is positioned inside a tree trunk, with the adult gorilla watching closely. A cobra is wrapped in the tree above, with his head lingering above the gorillas. The alligator is positioned in front of the tree, also glaring toward the gorillas. A fence separates the alligator from the others. The child says about the scene:

> "The baby monkey is hiding in his house from the alligator. The fence is keeping the alligator out, but the baby is still scared, and she doesn't want to leave. The mommy monkey says she wants the baby to come out and play, but the baby is too scared. She doesn't know it, but there is even a snake above her just waiting for her to come out."

In this scene, the following themes may be noted: negative initial content, negative final content (no resolution), no emotional shift, danger, neediness (mommy monkey wants baby to come out, but does not offer help to remove fear), and labeling of emotions. If the baby monkey is the Self-toy, Self-representations are judged to be inactive and frozen. There is a lack of confidence in self-efficacy and a clear fear of the unknown. Similarly, "Other" Object representations include an attentive, but passive mother figure. The therapist may respond by discussing some of these themes with the child by asking or "wondering" about the characters in the scene. You may say, for example:

> "That baby gorilla looks so scared it's like she can't do anything. She's afraid of the alligator, and even though she doesn't know the snake is there, she's afraid it might be. So I bet she thinks it's just safer to stay

inside where nothing can hurt her. Hmmmm? I wonder how she will ever feel okay with all of these things out there."

You may then follow up by saying, "Hey, I have an idea about what we can do with this alligator. I have a cage that it can't get out of it. Let's put it in that where it can't get to the baby. [You put the alligator in a cage.] There, now the baby is safe from the alligator. Now, what about this snake though? What can we do with it?"

In this case, the child is given a chance to decide what to do about the snake. If she does not come up with a solution, you may offer some options (e.g., the snake can be baited away with a tasty treat, the mother gorilla beats up the snake, a blanket is placed over its eyes so it can't see, etc.). In some cases, the child may decline all options, as a way of communicating a sense of hope-lessness. If this occurs, you should take an emotion-focused, rather than pro-blem-focused approach, and empathize with the baby gorilla's predicament and construct a "container" for the baby's emotions ("Whew, it feels like there are some things no one can fix. That sure must be hard. No wonder baby needs her mommy close by! Does mommy know how hard it is for baby to feel like that? I wonder if baby just needs a hug from mommy, instead of being asked to come out. Maybe if mommy holds her long enough, baby will start to feel safe again."). This intervention, or some similar variant, is con-structed to communicate an understanding of the intensity of the child's fear and a willingness to help her figure out how to manage a feeling of such intensity. **It is often necessary early in therapy**, before a child has learned coping skills or been able to internalize some of the therapeutic interventions, **to acknowledge that fear cannot always be eliminated, but that, over time, the child can expect to find hope in being able to manage and cope with it**.

Closing the session

To close the session, review the session with the child. Review how you talked about several types of feelings, both positive ones and scary ones. Highlight that the point of the play was to show how feelings are important, and worth paying attention to. Also highlight that feelings have different levels and that it is important to be able to tell the difference between "small" feelings and "big" feelings.

Session 3 – Somatic anxiety

Purpose

To review and elaborate distinguishing anxious feelings from other types of feelings. To learn more about somatic responses to anxiety. To introduce relaxation training (through play).

Goals

1   Help the child become aware of different signs of anxiety
2   Help child relax
3   Help child relax in an anxious situation

A major focus in this session is to elicit discussion about somatic and physiological symptoms of anxiety. Hence, a scene is introduced which is designed to provoke fear in most children. Even if children do not respond to the scene with fear, they will intuitively understand that fear is an expected response to the scene. This scene contains only a single story stem. In nearly all cases in FELT trials, the story stem used in this session takes the entire session. Children will also vary in their pre-existing understanding of physiological signs of anxiety. Some children may, with little help, be able to share exactly what happens in their body when they are scared; others may need more structure and more help. For capturing physiological signs of anxiety, it is okay to play this scene by ear and to supplement suggestions as needed to teach the child about what happens in a person's body when they are afraid. A few of the most important "symptoms" to list include heart beating faster, feeling short of breath, and muscle activation (feeling tight or feeling loose, like "jelly"), as these will tie in most closely to activities introduced in session 4 when teaching relaxation. However, any additional physiological symptoms may be added.

Occasionally, children may list symptoms that aren't commonly tied to human anxiety – "My nose feels twitchy" – or symptoms that don't make much sense – "My knees felt like clowns!" Therapists should usually avoid negating these symptoms. They should not say things like, "That doesn't sound like anxiety." Instead, it is preferable to just accept what the child reports. What is important here is that the child makes a connection between anxiety and several physiological manifestations. If some of these manifestations are "non-traditional," it is acceptable to just "roll with it." In the example of symptoms that don't make sense, you can seek clarification. In the case of the child whose "knees felt like clowns," he remembered seeing a clown who did a "falling" bit at a birthday party, where the clown would fall over dramatically to make kids laugh. So, when he said his knees felt like clowns, he meant that he felt like falling over.

Activity 1: Signs of worry

Introduction: "Do you remember last time we played about times when kids have different feelings like happy, excited, and worried [insert any other emotions played with particular child]? Today, we are going to do some more of that. I have another idea for a story to get us started."

Note: the following scene is meant to elicit an obvious and strong sense of fear, using a home burglary. Though usually children respond well to it, therapists should exercise caution if the scene is too similar to any occurrences in the child's real life or if the child has shown a strong negative reaction to past attempts at confronting fear within therapy. In those cases, such a scene may be better withheld until later in treatment, as a targeted stem, and this scene can be replaced with a different, less "familiar" fear-eliciting stem.

Story: Robbers.

Toys needed: child, two robbers, two parents, chair, computer, valuables (e.g., money, jewelry, art, artifacts, etc.), thieves' kit (in FELT development, this included a bag with a grappling hook, crowbar, fishing pole (which is used to fish valuables out while avoiding security measures), weapons, and a car which thieves could use to escape with valuables once stolen). Ideally, you should also be prepared with police/superheroes which may be used to capture robbers and cages/fences as makeshift jails, but generally these toys are not set up in the beginning, especially if the child is already aware they exist and can request them if desired. They are instead among the general inventory of all toys available during all sessions.

Story stem: If a play house with at least two rooms is available, it should be used for this story. If no such house is available, partitions are placed to create two rooms. In one room, a chair is set up in front of a computer. In the other room, place valuables. To start, the parents are standing next to each other, and both are facing the child. All are standing within the room with the computer. In this example, we are assuming the child has chosen a girl as the child figure.

Key: D = Dad, M = Mom, C = Child, R1 = Robber 1, R2 = Robber 2, N = Narrator

D: Okay honey, I'm going to work. You have a good day with Mom. [Dad leaves.]

C: Okay, bye Dad.

M: I'm going to go outside to work in the garden. You stay here and play on the computer. If you need something, just come out and get me. [Mom leaves. Girl is inside the house alone.]

N: Now the girl goes to play on the computer. After a little while, two robbers come in the other room to steal [whatever valuables are used]. They come in through a window, but they don't know the girl is just in the other room. When they start to go through things, the girl hears a noise [it helps to knock some things over, here]. What happens next?

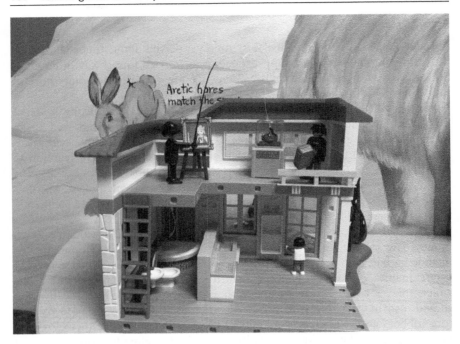

Fig. 8.3 Robbers breaking in upstairs during the Robber stem. In this example, the child is running outside to get help from her mother, who is outside working in the garden. Photo by author.

The child should now be allowed to finish the story. Respond appropriately as described throughout the manual. This particular play stem tends to elicit quite elaborate stories with multiple plot lines as children have fun with possible solutions to the robbery. Consequently, it generally works best for therapists to follow the child's lead for most of the story with regard to content, looking for themes and considering potential later responses to those themes, focusing on "assessment" more than intervention at least during the first play-through. Commentary should focus mainly on highlighting somatic aspects of situational anxiety/fear, but should be done so unobtrusively to the "flow" of play. For example, if an action-packed scene is happening, it is not necessary to pause the action to ask how or what a character is feeling. However, if there is a logical pause point to "check in," then it is permissible to do so. If a child seems stuck and unable to move the narrative forward, interventional suggestions can be offered to guide toward healthy resolution. Still, these are rarely necessary in a first play-through. Most children are able to engage with and complete the Robber stem on their own, and most do so with many details and drawn-out story lines. If a child does not engage well with the story and resolves it quickly, you may consider adding some intrigue to draw it out on your own. For example, if the robbers are immediately arrested, put into jail, and all valuables recovered, you may consider having the robbers break out of jail and then see how the child responds. Similarly, if the child has the robbers kill everyone inside and get away with all the valuables without a trace, the therapist may introduce a super-detective who makes it his life's mission to capture the bad guys and bring them to justice.

After a first play-through with the Robber stem, there are usually several unanswered questions or unresolved components. For example, the robbers may get captured, but the child's fear and "trauma" of the incident are ignored. You will usually need to go back to parts of this story after it is completed and reassess and/or intervene as necessary. During a second play-through, interventional components are much heavier-handed. With a more assessment-focused play-through in your pocket, you can now intervene more purposefully to address whatever the child could not resolve on their own in the first play-through. Hence, it is fairly typical for therapists to revisit parts of the Robber stem or the stem in its entirety to help address anything left "hanging" in thematic analysis.

In my experience, children often also return to the Robber stem multiple times in later sessions too. It is a clear favorite among children who've received FELT and offers quite a bit of rich material for children to explore a variety of fears.

Note: it is hoped that the child will be able to identify some signs of fear in the girl. Regardless of how the girl responds (she may flee in terror, call for her mom, call the police, or beat up the robbers all on her own), you should attempt to elicit some reference to the girl's bodily experience of anxiety that occurred before, during, and after her response. You should also help the child differentiate these feelings from those associated with happiness or excitement (as played in earlier sessions). Lastly, you should work to introduce some basic ideas to resolve the fear (e.g., getting help from a parent/adult, reminding themselves they are safe and robbers can't hurt them anymore).

Detailed examples and analysis of potential resolutions to the Robber stem were explored in Chapter 2. Generally speaking, though, the Robber stem has proven to be an excellent means for evaluating early depictions of the child's Self, largely because this is the first stem where the child character is purposefully left alone. Even though a parent is nearby, the child must navigate a rather difficult situation at least temporarily on their own. Thus, the way the child responds to this challenge will often reflect key aspects of the Self, particularly self-competence. So, therapists are encouraged to be alert to potential aspects of the Self displayed in the Robber stem, which can then be used as part of the overall case conceptualization.

[OPTIONAL] Activity 2: Child-specific anxiety story

Though it is rare for children to have enough time in this session for an additional story, some do complete the Robber stem more quickly than others, in which case there can be some time left over in session. If this occurs, activity 2 invites children to create a story of their own about anxiety. The goal and format then are identical to activity 2.3.[2]

Interventions as described previously may be used as necessary during this process. *Additional* questions to ask may be:

1   Does the child in this story feel the same, better, or worse than the child in the robber story? (This helps the client begin to differentiate between different levels of anxiety.)
2   How does the child know if she has "too much" anxiety? Or when it is "not too bad"? (This helps the child begin to delineate which levels of the hierarchy are manageable and which are not.)
3   How does the child calm down? Or how does the child keep the anxiety from getting "too much"?

    a   Within this realm, you may make suggestions for how the child can calm.

Closing remarks

Before the close of the session, the child should be notified that the next meeting will be held between the parents and you, but that this will not replace the child's time with you. The child is informed that this process is designed so that you can teach the parents how they can help the child too. You should also tell the child that they may expect the parents to participate in some joint sessions at some point as well, so that the parents can learn even better about how to help. You should gauge the child's reaction to this possibility and answer any questions she may have about what role the parents may play (the parent component of FELT is outlined in Chapter 9).

In between sessions 3 and 4

You will meet with parents for the parent-only session between sessions 3 and 4. The outline and purpose for this session are described in Chapter 9.

Session 4

Purpose

To introduce relaxation training. To review somatic cues that show the child is anxious.

Goals

1   Acknowledge parent session
2   Review somatic feelings of anxiety, with a focus on muscle tension
3   Teach relaxation through symbolic play

This session is structured differently than others so far. There will still be playful activities, and storytelling methods will still be employed. However, this session, you will use theatrical (role-playing) or puppet-based play, rather than toy-based play. Choosing the method of play will depend largely on the age of the child and on their own preferences, and toy-based play is not prohibited if neither theatrical nor puppet-based play seems to work. However, there is a benefit to teaching children how to use non-toy-based play therapeutically, in that children in their daily lives will not always have access to toys when needing to cope with anxiety. Thus, engaging children in alternative forms of play helps generalize their ability to learn and use skills when toys are not available. Furthermore, activities 4.2 and 4.3 will be repeated in subsequent sessions throughout the rest of FELT, usually prior to initiation of toy-based play. Thus, teaching kids these non-toy-based relaxation skills helps facilitate their expedient repetition in future sessions. In other words, the activity can be repeated in future sessions quickly, without needing to set up toys or play scenes, therefore allowing more time to complete other planned session activities in future sessions.

Given these considerations, you should set up the room for session 4 differently than in previous sessions. In sessions 1–3, therapists have usually already prepared the room with toys that were going to be used in the sessions, and play usually centered around a general play area (i.e., a table), which helped structure the sessions. In this session, you should not start with any toys "out." Rather, toys should be put away at onset of session. Furthermore, it is useful to create a large space in the room for movement, if possible. Children are likely to notice this and may begin to wonder where the toys are. It is important, then, to be prepared to start quickly with activities 4.1 and 4.2, so that you can engage the child efficiently in session before they begin to search for toys. You will alert them early that you will use a different type of play today. Lastly, if you are working in a room where there is insufficient area for movement and "exercise," as outlined in activity 4.2, you may wish to plan an alternative area (e.g., hallway or stairwell) for engaging in the activity, after which you can return to your reserved therapy room/office.

Activity 1: Talking about the parent session

Briefly tell the child you met with the parent(s) as planned and offer a brief, developmentally appropriate summary of the exchange. Explain that today the parents are going to be invited for the end of the session so that you and the child can show and tell them the story you create today. Tell the child that the story will be about relaxing and that it would be good for the parents to know it so that they can help the child practice at home. Invite and respond to questions appropriately.

Activity 2: Physiological reactivity

Introduction: "You might have noticed that things look different in our office today. Today we are going to do something different. In the past, we played with toys to make stories and scenes about different things to learn about feelings and anxiety. This time, we'll do some different, fun things. To start, remember how last week we talked about what happens in your body when you get scared? [Review these lessons from last session as needed, by asking the child to recite again what can happen in a person's body when they are afraid. Be sure to include increased heart rate and breathing harder, among any other symptoms listed. Once you have reviewed these, continue with the following script.] Well, you know, there are other things we can do to make our bodies do those same things, and sometimes we can use that to help practice relaxing our bodies. For example, to make our hearts beat faster and breathe a little harder, we can do some exercise, or do a silly dance, or something like that. What do you say we try that out, now? What would you like to do together?"

You may choose to exercise with the child by doing jumping jacks, running in circles, doing push-ups, sit-ups, etc. You may also perform a silly dance with the child or do some other lively activity. Only do the activity long enough to produce a noticeable physiological change. Usually, one to two minutes is enough to produce a change. If you are unable to participate in these activities with the child due to physical or health reasons, you may simply watch the child. If the child is unable to perform these activities for physical or health reasons, you may choose other activities as listed in Table 8.2 below. It is not advised that you do the activity and have the child watch, as part of the main reasons for this activity is to boost the child's ability to monitor and control their own physiology.

Some therapists familiar with treatments for anxiety disorders may recognize that this activity is a form of interoceptive exposure. Interoception is a person's sense of the internal state of their body, that is, their relative ability to recognize internal cues. Like with all senses, some are more sensitive than others in their interoception. For example, some children can go hours and hours without recognizing they are hungry and have not eaten or that they

Table 8.2 Interoceptive exposure activities for children and anxiety symptoms each is designed to mimic

Activity	Physiological target	Suggested time limit	Comment
Running, jumping jacks, push-ups, sit-ups, any other exercise	Increase heart rate and breathing rate; muscle tightness/ fatigue	One to two minutes. Two to three minutes for exceptionally fit children	Feel free to switch exercises as needed/ desired.
Overbreathing (breathe forcefully, fast and deep, as if hyperventilating)	Shortness of breath; hyperventi-lation and other panic breathing	30–60 seconds	Consider additional infection control pro-cedures as needed to reduce risk of disease transmission from forceful breathing.
Breathing through a straw (hold nose and breathe through a drinking straw, at a regular pace)	Shortness of breath; labored breathing	30–90 seconds	Consider additional infection control procedures as needed (e.g., point the straw into a cup)
Hold breath	Shortness of breath; labored breathing	Max hold	
Spin in circles as fast as possible	Dizziness; lightheadedness	20–60 seconds	If standing, be pre-pared to sit afterward for stability.
Shake head from side to side, with eyes open	Dizziness; light-headedness (mild)	20–60 seconds	This tends to produce a milder sensation of dizziness and may not work well for kids with a high dizziness tolerance.
Put head between legs and sit up quickly; repeat in rapid succession	Head rush; lightheadedness	30–60 seconds	Exercise caution in children prone to orthostatic hypoten-sion, so that they don't faint from this procedure.
Head banging. Put on some (clean) hard rock music and rock out!	Head rush; lightheadedness	30–120 seconds	This is just a fun var-iation on the other head rush techniques. Many kids like to pretend to head bang as they rock out.

Activity	Physiological target	Suggested time limit	Comment
"Hulk mode" – tense all body muscles and push pulse pressure toward the face, as if lifting a heavy weight with improper form/ breathing	Increase blood pressure; muscle tightness; head rush; seeing "stars"	10–15 seconds	This will cause a sharp, brief rise in blood pressure; check with medical provider to ensure this is safe.
Arm wrestling	Increase blood pressure; muscle tightness; increase breathing rate	Two minutes	Make this challenging for the child. Don't let them win without a fight. Make them work hard and give all they've got to beat you.
Dance party	Increase heart rate and breathing rate; muscle fatigue	Two to three minutes	Choose a favorite danceable song and break out your best moves.

need to urinate but have not peed. This can be considered a form of insensitive interoception. Others can be hypersensitive to interoceptive cues. They notice every little thing that happens in their body, which may cause anxiety, especially somatic or hypochondriacal anxiety. Most people are more sensitive to some cues than to others (e.g., they notice potty needs, but not hunger needs or they notice stomach aches but not changes in heart rate). Like any interoceptive exposure, this activity is designed to help children 1) build interoceptive skill for noticing mild physiological symptoms of anxiety, and 2) reduce distress about what those symptoms mean or what they may become. The next activity (activity 4.3) is designed to take the next step of then giving children a skill to use to regain control over their physiological reactions and use playful mindfulness skills to selectively focus attention away from the symptoms, so that they can more easily return to baseline. Table 8.2 below lists several interoceptive exposure activities that can be used as part of this activity in this session (and in future sessions, when the activity is repeated).

An important part of this activity is teaching children to monitor and track their own physiological reactions. Typically, I have done this through "low-tech" methods by asking children to count their heart rate[3] using a stethoscope or by simply feeling their pulse with their fingers and counting. Stethoscopes are used because children usually find them fun and interesting, as most children do not use stethoscopes regularly in their daily lives. Thus, they are intrigued by how they work and enjoy having a chance to listen to their own (and/or your) heartbeats through the stethoscope. If a child is wearing a fitness watch that automatically tracks their heart rate (which has become more common in the last half decade or so than it was when FELT was originally created), it is advised that they still engage in their own counting process, not relying on the watch to inform them of changes in heart rate. Counting their own heart rate helps children learn how to recognize and monitor their own bodies for subtle physiological indicators of anxiety, which they then learn to control through relaxation. Using an automated digital monitor, when not paired with self-monitoring, detracts from this learning process. Typically, I ask children to count their heart rate for 30 seconds, and then I multiply by two to get a better bpm count. Doubling the number this way allows for a larger variation between the pre- and post-relaxation counts (see below), which can be more meaningful for children.

It is **not** imperative that children *accurately* count their own heart rates during this activity. In fact, in FELT studies and in clinical experience, most younger children are actually quite inaccurate at counting their own heart rates, and it is common after a bout of exercise for them to report they only counted 30 beats per minute (or, to the contrary, they report a ridiculously high number, like 200 bpm). It is for this reason that I do *not* recommend children collect baseline readings of heart rate prior to the activity. There is no need to count heart rate before exercise/physiological arousal. Rather, it works better for the first count to come *after* the arousing activity. What we have found repeatedly is that children intuitively understand, partially because you have told them as much, that their heart rate should decrease after the relaxation activity. Thus, once you perform the relaxation activity (4.3) and then remeasure heart rate, almost all children will report a lower count than the post-arousal count, even if it is impossibly slow (e.g., 15 bpm). As therapist, you should not concern yourself with the accuracy of heart rate measurements made by the child. Rather, your primary objective is to ensure the child understands and reports that relaxation activities also relax heart rate.

Activity 3: Relaxing

Now, you will start the process of helping the child relax from their artificially induced, hyperaroused state. You can use any evidence-based relaxation method for this activity, but the suggested activity is designed to maintain the narrative nature of FELT and to adapt mindfulness/meditation skills to the playful nature of children. As outlined in Chapter 7, a major goal of this session is to help kids learn ways to achieve behavioral sedation/de-arousal.

Introduction: "Alright, now that we've got our hearts beating faster and our lungs working harder, our bodies are doing exactly what they do when we get scared or worried. Now we can practice telling a story to help get our bodies relaxed again. This story is going to be about relaxing. Let's make up a story about being happy and calm and relaxed. First, let's figure out where to set the story? Where should we go in our minds for this story?"

It is common, especially early in FELT, for children to struggle to independently tell a therapeutic story. Thus, in this case, your focus as therapist is to teach through modeling and interactive storytelling how to formulate a therapeutic story. It is advised to begin with a setting. This story will best serve its purpose if it is individualized to the client. Therefore, no stems or examples are provided here. Each child should have his or her own idea about what constitutes a happy, relaxing, or calm scene. As therapist, you should work with the child to develop a story that is relaxing for them. So, in choosing a setting, the child is often instructed to select a place that makes them happy, and suggestions can be offered if the child hesitates. Some therapists make verbal suggestions – "What do you think? Should we go to the woods? The mountains? The beach? An amusement park? Your bedroom?" Other therapists may wish to utilize a "flipbook" of pictures that show relaxing or fun places. In providing options, it is important to remember that what we find relaxing as adults may be very different than what kids find relaxing. Whereas we may like to imagine rocking in a hammock on a serene beach preparing to take a glorious nap, kids may prefer a sprint through the woods chasing animals and stumbling upon an ice cream stand run by a squirrel. So, it is important to follow the child's lead in creating this story and to not focus heavily on whether the content of the story seems relaxing or not. The therapeutic effect of this activity is rarely found in the imagination of a relaxing scene, but rather in mindful redirection from an anxious stimulus toward a fun story. In other words, if using this skill in real-time to manage anxious thoughts, there is still quite a bit of therapeutic benefit in the child being able to refocus their mind on the story, even if the story is ridiculous and not "relaxing" in a traditional sense, rather than on the thing they are worrying about. Establishing skill and mindful mental redirection is an important first step in preparing the Self to battle and take on anxiety.

Although the child leads the content of the story, the therapist usually takes an active role in asking relevant questions to keep the story going and to mark the details of the mindful activity. As is commonly used in mindful meditations, kids are encouraged to incorporate all five major senses – sight, smell, hearing, taste, and touch – into their story. At first, this is done rather surreptitiously. You do not need to instruct the child up front to try to incorporate all the senses. During the first story (this activity) it often works best to more furtively guide the child through the senses through questioning. So, once a location is established, you may ask the child first to describe what they see, and help them do so in great detail. Once a visual scene is set, you can ask about the temperature or the weather, which incorporates tactile senses. Next, you can search for opportunities to include smell. If the child mentions a flower, you can demonstrate picking a flower and smelling it, and then offer that flower for the child to smell too. Ask them what it smells like. Smells don't need to always be pleasant. Occasionally when telling fun stories, children may pretend a character has passed gas, which presents a useful opportunity to bring smell into the story. Food is also a useful story addition, as it adds both smell and taste. Experienced therapists often find interesting ways to suggest food-based additions to the story. Lastly, auditory experiences are frequent and easy to enhance by simply asking the child what they hear. Continue the story for around five minutes or so, or longer if desired, up to ten minutes. If necessary (due to time), help the child conclude the story by asking, "How should this story end?"

At the end of the story, first return to heart rate. Have the child remeasure their heart rate and notice any changes or decreases in heart rate. Ask the child about their experience – whether they feel different now than they did just before the story, what feels different, and so on. Most children intuitively understand and note a more relaxed state than what they felt after exercise. Even if they do not note a clear, drastic change in heart rate, they can at least note other signs that indicate they are more rested than they were immediately after the previous activity.

If necessary, you can also manipulate the counting period to help ensure that children get a lower count in heart rate compared to the post-exercise/pre-relaxation count. For example, if a child appears to be counting rapidly and you feel they may reach or exceed their pre-relaxation count, you may consider pausing, measuring with them, and counting aloud together at a slower pace. Alternatively, you can abbreviate the counting period (e.g., count for 20 seconds instead of 30) to get fewer beats. Many young children (those who are most likely to count inaccurately) will not be able to tell the difference between 20 seconds and 30 seconds, and in this case a small amount of harmless deception can help solidify the point of the activity, which is to note that heart rate will slow down if you relax. As a final measure, if there is no appreciable change in heart rate counts, you can suggest an additional relaxation period and instruct the child to see if a second trial slows down the heart rate more. Again, for most children, this suggestion is usually enough to tell them that the post-relaxation count is supposed to be lower than the post-exercise count, and they will adjust their own count accordingly. Often, this "placebo" affect is useful therapeutically to help children build confidence (self-efficacy) in their ability to manage anxiety. In other words, if they *believe* they can relax heart rate and other physiology by telling a relaxing story, they will be more likely to actually use it in managing anxiety.

Some astute children may also "catch on" that the reason they are more relaxed after the story is not necessarily due to the story itself, but to the passage of time and the body naturally returning to homeostasis. In these cases, children are reminded of the metaphor of the activity. In this activity, exercise is meant to represent something that causes children anxiety. By stopping exercise and replacing with relaxation, we are mimicking the same skill to be used for anxiety. You stop anxiety and replace with relaxation, just like you stopped exercise and replaced it with a story. Remind the child that exercise is used as a way to *practice* the skill and to show the child they have control over their body. Just like they can control here when they exercise and when they relax, they can do the same with anxiety. Furthermore, they learn to notice the signs of anxiety and how they can use relaxation skills to get those signs to return to baseline.

Note: this entire activity can use simple verbal storytelling techniques, which have been shown to work well for the majority of children. Occasionally, some children do like to "act out" the scene in dramatic fashion, which is allowed. Still, since this activity is repeated every session from here, therapists are advised to try at least on occasion to encourage the child to tell a "verbal"/imagination-only story, without acting it out. This suggestion is made so that the child has well-balanced coping skills that can be used in a variety of settings. An imagined story can be told anywhere at (almost) any time with very little to no disruption. If, for example, a child has test anxiety at school, being skilled at telling a relaxing story in their head (without props or without acting it out) can help them actually use the skill at school, just before a test.

Activity 4: Progressive muscle relaxation story

Activity 3 focused on cognitive relaxation measures. Activity 4 helps teach an adjunctive skill, progressive muscle relaxation (PMR), in a kid-friendly way. We do this by transitioning to a different activity and a different story. In this next activity, the child will tell another relaxation story, following a similar method and style as activity 3. However, this time, they will do so in response to a worry stem, which can help solidify the technique's use as a response to anxiety. Furthermore, in this activity, *after telling the relaxation story*, children will be taught how to use PMR to attenuate residual anxiety. You will start with a seamless transition from activity 3.

Introduction: "Alright, super job. A few minutes ago, we were all worked up. Our hearts were racing, our blood was pumping hard, and [any other signs mentioned]. Then, we did the relaxing story and everything went back to normal. That's pretty cool. I wonder if we can do the same thing when you feel worried to help relax. This time, I'm going to make up a story about 'Worrying William' [or 'Worrying Wendy,' depending on your preference]. It will work a lot like when we use toys, but this time, we'll just use our words instead. I'll start the story, and then I'll ask you to finish it. Ready?"

Next, you will tell a story that sets up your client into a scenario that has been revealed as being an anxious situation for the child. The story should utilize symbolic fantasy and should follow the same procedures as any other therapeutic narrative used in FELT. Three example stories are provided after this session as guidelines. Each was written for and used with children who participated in the treatment development study. If you are a beginner, you may use one of the sample stories, but you are encouraged to choose or create a story with as close a relevance to a real problem for your client as possible.

After the story, you should ask the child, "Do you have any ideas how William/Wendy might calm down?" Hopefully, the child may suggest using the relaxation story created earlier. If the child does not spontaneously make this suggestion, you may lead the child toward that idea (i.e., "Remember that story we told earlier about relaxing?"). Once the child mentions the relaxation story, tell them, "That's a good idea. I bet he *could* do that. Let's tell another relaxation story for William." Then, repeat either the same or a different relaxation story as in the previous activity.

After the relaxation story is told, introduce the idea of PMR. Say, "I think William feels almost relaxed now, but I think he needs one thing. Did you know that sometimes when people worry too much, their muscles get all tight without them even knowing it? I wonder if we can make up a story or a game that will help William loosen up a little. Do you have any ideas? [Allow response. Some kids may suggest some stretches, or yoga, or other relevant muscle-relaxation activity, all of which could be included in this activity.] If not, I have one. It's called 'Righty Tighty, Lefty Loosey.' Do you know how to play?"

You may then teach the child how to play. Righty Tighty, Lefty Loosey involves a systematic effort to first tighten muscles on the right side of the body while keeping those on the left loose and relaxed (and then switching after a count to five). With each muscle, you alternately tighten and loosen each side for a five-count each time. The game is for two (or more) players, and players take turns calling out a muscle to be tightened. The game can become fun/difficult by calling out muscles that are difficult to contract (e.g., ears). As you play the game, it is important to use common principles from other approaches to PMR, such as alerting the child to attend to the alternating sensations of strain and release and to how the child can exert control over the release through purposeful muscle relaxation.

After the game, review the reasons for the game and how it may be used therapeutically when indicated. **Be sure to emphasize that the game helps the child learn how to *relax* certain muscles, which they may need to do when feeling anxious.** With some children, it may be particularly helpful to use imagery regarding their somatic symptoms. So, a child who gets "knots in her stomach" when nervous can practice "untying the knots" with her stomach muscles. Similarly, that child may "catch the butterflies" in her stomach using her stomach muscles. Some children even enjoy counting the butterflies as they catch them.

Activity 5: Parents

To close the session, invite the parents to join you and allow the child to share their relaxation story and the "Righty Tighty, Lefty Loosey" game with the parents. Be sure to cover the reasons/indications for the techniques and encourage the parents to help the child practice the techniques at home or with friends. Practice the activities briefly with parents in the room.

Worrying William/Wendy story stems

Storms

Wendy was a little girl who loved being outside. She loved to lie outside and look at the clouds. She loved to pick flowers and smell them. And she especially loved playing in the rain. She loved to run around in her bright yellow raincoat, to feel the water run down her cheeks, and to splash in the mud puddles with her rain boots. One day, Wendy was sitting inside coloring a picture, and it began to sprinkle outside. Getting excited, Wendy jumped up from her seat and asked her mom if she could play outside. Her mom said that she could, as long as she put on her rain clothes first. So Wendy put on all her rain clothes: her big yellow jacket, her yellow hat, her old muddy pants, and her striped boots, and then she ran outside to play.

As she was playing outside, the rain began to pick up – it started raining harder. Dark, scary-looking clouds moved in, and the wind started blowing really hard. Wendy didn't mind though, this just meant she could have more fun playing in puddles. She splashed in puddles and stood under the rain. She even stuck out her tongue to catch the big, giant raindrops that were now falling. Then, Wendy started hearing thunder, and the wind started blowing *really* hard. Wendy's mom opened the door and shouted, "Wendy! Get inside now. There's a tornado coming!" Wendy immediately felt scared. [Use this as an opportunity to ask the child, "What did being scared feel like?" and allow a response.] Wendy ran inside and her mom said, "Come on, let's get in the hallway, away from windows." Wendy and her mom hid in the hallway. That's when Wendy REALLY started getting worried. All that time, she was thinking _____ [work with the child to fill in the blank with some worried thoughts].

Do you have any ideas about how Wendy can relax?

Sports/Performance anxiety

Note: details may be changed to be made more appropriate for different kinds of sports.

Wendy was a little girl who loved to dance. She loved turning, spinning, and twirling, and jumping, and bouncing, and running on her tippy toes, and all the other things that little girls do when they dance. She even liked the cute little outfits that little dancers wear. Her big sister was a dancer, and she saw her sister perform on stage and thought it was so beautiful. So, she wanted to learn how to dance like that. Wendy decided to join a class to help her learn how to dance better. She asked her mom if she could sign up, and mom said that she could. So, mom took her to visit a dance studio where she could take a class with other girls her age. Wendy was so excited at first because she knew that she would soon be getting to do something she loved.

On Wendy's first day of class, she met some of the other girls, and they talked before class. Wendy thought they were all really nice, and she even made friends with some of them. Then, the class started, and the teacher was really nice too. She smiled a lot and was a really good helper with all the girls in the class. She even gave extra help to Wendy, since it was her first day and all. As Wendy was learning how to do all the moves, she began to notice that she wasn't as good as the other girls. She couldn't do some of the moves they could. Still, she kept trying and finished the class. After the class was over, the teacher told her that she did a good job, and Wendy smiled.

Still, she worried that she wasn't as good as the others, and she thought that maybe some of the other girls' moms who were watching the class were thinking that Wendy wasn't very good. Next week, when it came time for class again, Wendy felt kind of funny in her tummy. She felt like it was tying itself in knots. She was really nervous. She almost felt like throwing up. ["Why was her tummy acting like that?" – allow a response from the child.] She told her mom she didn't feel well, and her mom didn't know what was wrong. She told her mom, "I feel nervous," and mom knew that Wendy must be nervous about her new class. Mom wanted to help Wendy relax.

Do you have any ideas about how Wendy can relax?

Test anxiety

Once upon a time, a boy named William wanted to be an astronaut. He loved to fly, and he wanted to see the Earth from space. One day, he went to space camp, and he LOVED it. They had space shuttles for him to get in and a little spacesuit for him to wear. It was AWESOME. Then, at the end, the grown-ups that worked at the camp told William how hard it was to become an astronaut and that he would have to take lots of tests. They even had a test for him to take right then and there that would say if he would be a good astronaut or not. But William HATED tests [blech!]! He was always afraid he would do badly on the test, and he would get so nervous that he could never think of the answers, even to the easy questions that he knew the answers to the night before. William started to feel butterflies in his stomach [you should use child-specific somatic symptoms] because he knew he would fail this test and never become an astronaut.

Do you have any ideas about how William might relax?

In between sessions 4 and 5

Case conceptualization, with an example

You may recall that in FELT development studies, therapists being trained in FELT were asked after session 4 to prepare a case conceptualization to be discussed in fidelity monitoring sessions. So, if you have not done so already, you may choose at this point to prepare a working case conceptualization for yourself, following the FELT model. By now, and based on the information you've gathered so far in treatment, you should have a fair idea of the various propagating, manifest, and temporal factors that affect your client. Keeping these in mind as you prepare for ongoing sessions will help you respond as therapeutically as possible to expressed needs in session.

In particular, FELT focuses heavily on the psychodynamic propagating factors mentioned in Chapter 6. So, it can help to ask yourself what unmet needs seem most prominent so far in therapy. For example, let's imagine Steve is an eight-year-old boy who presented for treatment with generalized anxious distress. He completed the Spilled juice stem as offered in the example previously, where he depicts punitive, misattuned parents, and extreme fear of "getting in trouble." Let's say he also completed the Robber stem by having the robbers kidnap him and take him to their secret hideout. While kidnapped, Steve plans a way of escape and, in doing so, captures the bad guys, and they are taken to jail. In his "Happy time" story, Steve created an endearing moment of sitting on his couch, snuggling with parents, watching a movie together, and eating popcorn and candy. In creating an anxiety story, Steve placed some animals in a jungle scene and separated the animals by prey or predator. He then started a war between them, which the prey animals lost miserably, save one, a little lamb who hid in the bushes until the fight was over. After the predators left, he showed the lamb alone and scared, trying to save the dead animals, some of which he did revive, and some of which he didn't. Together, the revived animals worked to create a dam (a suggestion made by the therapist) between the two sides of the jungle which would keep the predators on their side forever. The scene ended with each group on their own side, and they never saw each other again. The prey animals rebuilt and started over.

Analyzing these various scenes for repeating themes, and focusing on potential psychological needs being expressed through play, we see a few standout needs:

1   There are repeated themes expressing fear of harm to the Self, that is, analgesia/comfort needs. In the Spilled juice stem, Steve fears punishment, a form of harm to the Self. In the Robber stem, Steve is kidnapped, and even though he made it out okay, there is an emotional shift that suggests he was likely at some point worried about what would happen to him (if he weren't worried, why would he escape, and why would he have the robbers arrested?). In the Happy time scene, Steve expresses needs being met. In this case, he is comfortable at home, doing an enjoyable activity, and free from the worry of any pain. In the jungle scene, the war shows great harm to the prey animals. Again, even though the harm was mostly undone and resolved in the play (through therapist intervention), there was still a clear expression of a fear of harm.

2   Steve seems especially concerned about separation of families, with hints of both loss of love and loss of Object anxiety. In the Spilled juice stem, disapproval from parents could be considered a loss of love anxiety. Kicking the dog and running off to his room is an active separation from his parent Objects; he's getting away from them, and though in the moment this is meant to be protective (to escape the situation), it also represents a distressing separation from parental figures, and it says a lot about his Object-relations. Being kidnapped in the Robber stem is another separation, as is being left as the sole survivor of the jungle war. Furthermore, in the Happy scene, he is together with family, suggesting a value for closeness and nurturance.

3   Steve seems to see himself as capable of taking care of problems when he needs to, especially if he can keep calm and stay safe long enough to escape the worst danger. Twice, Steve waited until he was alone to solve a problem. When kidnapped, he waited until the robbers were distracted and the worst of the danger had passed. He was in a cage, yes, but the worse danger had passed, allowing him to create a plan to escape. In the jungle, he hid until danger had passed, and then worked to help remedy the situation. So, Steve is telling you that when he is given a proper opportunity to do so, he believes he can solve really big problems. He just needs to establish enough safety/security to be able to work.

This example is a subtle form of disintegration anxiety. Steve's Self-image as a competent, active problem-solver is conditioned upon whether or not his environment allows him to be this person. When stress is too high (i.e., during the immediacy of the kidnapping and the war), his ability to problem solve falls apart. Instead, he freezes. Although this freezing does perhaps keep him safe in a way (especially during the war, where staying hidden kept him alive), it was not a conscious choice, but rather an automatic reaction driven by fear/anxiety. He did not "allow" himself to be kidnapped in order to accomplish a goal, nor did he actively seek a hiding place or reason that he should "stay hidden" to avoid danger. These things just happened as he was frozen by fear. Once that freezing passed, though, Steve could activate his more competent Self.

What we want, ideally, though, is for Steve to be able to activate this competent Self even in the face of great distress. We want consistency (integration) of this Self. We want him to decide to hide when hiding serves him, not to just "get lucky."

Although given Steve's age we would not expect him to achieve total Self-constancy, we can promote better Self-cohesion by helping him highlight how this competent, problem-solving Self can be controlled (by his ego) to emerge more adaptively.

Consulting Table 3.1 of this book, therapists can see that at eight years old, Steve is just transitioning from the middle childhood phase to the late childhood phase of Self-development. As such, it should not be too surprising that he still depicts himself in a generally positive light, and self-competence seems strong. However, they may still wonder how he sees himself in relation to peers, whether he can identify some core trait labels, and whether he has begun to incorporate societal standards into his vision of himself. Perhaps the therapist may recall some emerging trait language in how Steve depicted himself in play, in particular that he is "brave." He said this several times in both the Robber and the Jungle scenes. Still, there hasn't yet been a lot of material to more fully formulate if Steve values other traits along with bravery. So, the therapist may wish to specifically focus some future analyses to explore other traits Steve sees in himself.

Steve's therapist may also wonder if Steve can change his Self-depictions to fit realistic societal expectations. In the Robber and Jungle stems, Steve resolved scenes rather miraculously – some *deus ex machina* resolutions. So, the therapist may wonder if Steve can still respond so competently if he is restricted to respond in more realistic or socially plausible ways. Consequently, Steve's therapist may wish to consider some future play scenes that focus on putting him in situations he is more likely to face in his daily life, perhaps involving school pressures and peer relationships. We have some good ideas from early sessions about Steve's loss of Object and loss of love needs, but we don't know much about his popularity needs or how he manages tensions in his more "horizontal"[4] relationships. So, future play sessions and future analyses may hone toward this need.

Steve's depictions of caregivers show some distress, and there are some mild insinuations so far in play that Steve may even perceive some occasional role reversal with regard to his parents. In scenes of severe distress (Juice, Robber, and Jungle scenes), he has not yet at all shown that he feels he can rely on his parents to help him out when he needs it. This is abnormal in children Steve's age, where it is healthy for children to seek help from adults. So, Steve's therapist should also plan to continue to monitor his attitudes toward caregivers and should work to help Steve adjust his sense of security that caregivers can help solve problems. If real problems are noted in the parents' actual, real-world behaviors (explored in more depth during the parent session), Steve's therapist should recommend a plan for the parents to correct these problems. This may involve recommendations for individual therapy for the parents or adjunct family-based therapy for everyone, if needed. If parenting interventions are implemented, Steve's therapist can then monitor over time to see if Steve's depictions of caregivers in play are reliably moving toward healthier directions.

On the biological level, we will have heard at this point how Steve experiences his body in relation to anxiety and hyperarousal, and he has learned, in session 4, some concrete ways to de-escalate that physiological cascade when he needs to. We do not expect him to be skilled in this area yet, but moving forward we know that one goal of therapy is to help Steve experience an increased sense of control over his body. Some of this will be accomplished through ongoing practice of session 4 activities. Another portion will be highlighted through future play, using those same and similar skills in played characters to help them calm their physiology in response to anxiety.

Overall then, based on this conceptualization of Steve, some key therapeutic needs arise:

1   Steve needs to resolve his fear of pain/discomfort to an age-normative level. It is okay to want to avoid pain, but in Steve's case that avoidance seems to not always be serving him. In the Juice stem, he gets grounded and everything ends poorly. In the Robber stem, he gets kidnapped, when if he had run outside to mom for help right away, things may have gone better. Steve values being brave, and this is something the therapist can use to help him understand that bravery is not an avoidance of fear, but rather a decision to face fear.

2   Bravery is not the only key to fighting anxiety. Steve will need to develop other values of the Self that help him face his worries. Specifically, Steve's loss of love and loss of Object worry is unlikely to be resolved through bravery. Rather, he will need to see himself as "good enough," to know that love from Others is unconditional and won't be lost by mistakes he makes or other things he does wrong. He will need to develop a secure sense of Self that feels that he will always be good enough for his care-givers. Again, working with caregivers to teach them how to remind Steve that he is good enough will be paramount to meeting this goal.

3   Steve's therapist should conduct further evaluation to see if Steve's Object-relations with caregivers translate to other relationships, and then respond accordingly. Steve will also need to see himself as "good enough" for peers. He is entering an age where social peer relationships are likely to get more complicated, and it will benefit Steve to develop a consistent framework of himself within those relationships that can withstand those complexities.

4   Steve needs ongoing, active practice of cognitive and physiological skills to manage active anxiety when it arises.

For Steve, these goals would need to be integrated into the rest of FELT.

Session 5 – Self-talk and maladaptive thought patterns

Purpose

To review relaxation training. To focus intervening at the realm of Self-talk and maladaptive thought patterns.

Goals

1 Help reinforce child's ability to achieve relaxation
2 Help child identify anxiety-related thought patterns
3 Help child identify positive alternatives to anxiety-related thought patterns
4 Help child begin to gain mastery over anxious symptoms

In this session, you help the child transition from previous sessions which focused more heavily on somatic/physiological cues of anxiety, and you move toward a more cognitive realm. As outlined in the goals above, you will continue to review relaxation skills, but you will also add cognitive restructuring and "talking back" to anxious thoughts.

Activity 1: Physiology and relaxation review

Begin this session with another short, active exercise meant to stimulate physiological activity. This can be the same activity as last session, or can be a different one. Allow the child to choose. Immediately afterward, have the child develop another relaxation story as done before – it may be a different story or the same one. Alternatively, you and the child may play the "Righty Tighty, Lefty Loosey" game. The child may choose one or both. For time constraints, limit the entire process (physical stimulation plus relaxation) to approximately ten minutes. Remember to discuss how the child feels during each stage, highlighting physiological signs.

Activity 2: Vet visit

After activity 1, transition back to your usual play space (e.g., back to the table) and begin to introduce the next story stem. As you are getting toys together, inform the child that today you are going to play a scene where you work on worried thoughts and what things can be done to help worried thoughts when they come.
Toys needed: animal clinic, vet, dogs, people to serve as dogs' owners/families, vet supplies (medicines, casts, carts, etc.).

In this scene, you will be setting up a vet clinic with three dogs. Each dog will visit the vet in turn, and each will play a different role in enacting different levels of anxiety. The child can help you choose toys, and though we will use dogs in the description below, the child can choose other pets if they desire. You should instruct the child to choose three dogs and families for each dog. Next, you will instruct the child that in this scene, the dogs will be going to the vet, and each dog has a different level of worry about going. One dog is not worried at all. They feel very brave, and the vet doesn't scare them one bit. Another dog is a little bit nervous, but not too bad. The third dog is extremely nervous. The child can select which dog they want to play each role. Make a mental note of which is which and then proceed with the story stem as described in the example below.

Story stem: "Now let's play a story about three dogs who are sick. They are all going to the vet to find out what is wrong with them. The brown dog is very worried, the white dog is only a little worried, and the black dog is not worried at all. Each one goes to see the vet one at a time. Which one goes first?"

The child may then choose the order in which each dog goes to see the vet and should finish the story for each consecutive dog. If the child is unable to decide on an order, I recommend starting with the dog who is not scared at all, then the dog who is a little scared, then the dog who is very scared, as this order helps build comfort and skill with the scene gradually to maximize the chances the child will be able to use positive coping skills with the very scared dog. However, if the child chooses the very scared dog to go first, this can be allowed and interventions applied normally. Ask the child to complete the story, telling how each dog behaves throughout the vet visit and what is found to be wrong with each one. Invite the child to explore some of the somatic signs of the dogs. Also, inquire about the thoughts of each dog and monitor for positive or negative patterns. Based on the thoughts each dog has, respond in such a way as to highlight the state of worry of each dog. If necessary remind the child of the association. For example, you might say, "This is the dog who is *very* worried. I wonder what kinds of things this dog is thinking?" If the child does not readily make logical connections, you may help (perhaps by having the vet say, "This machine tells me what you're thinking, and it says you're so worried because you're thinking you might die. Is that right?" or, for the black dog, "You don't seem too worried at all. You must be thinking that everything is going to turn out okay."). The point is that the child uses the dogs to identify different levels of anxiety-related thinking, and the vet is available both to facilitate that process and to introduce and/or reinforce healthy thought patterns as necessary. Be sure to spend adequate time with each of the three dogs so that there are ample opportunities for the child to play about different strategies and approaches.

For the worried dogs, it is also important to follow other FELT principles to help provide intervention strategies to reduce distress. So, you may elect to highlight having family nearby as a social support, or allow the vet to administer a medicine that helps the dog not worry. After administration of these interventions, you should make a point to highlight the cognitive changes that occur through intervention. So, in response to social support, the dog might say/think, "I'm still scared, but I know my family wouldn't let anything bad happen to me, and I know I can trust they will take care of me." Alternatively, if the vet administers a medicine to help with worry, the dog may say/think, "Wow, I feel so much better. Now I'm thinking that everything will be okay and that I don't have to be afraid of the vet." Again, the main focus of this session is helping the child use play to identify worried thoughts and then to combat them in therapeutic ways, showing an understanding of active coping skills.

Generally, this vet visit activity can last 15–25 minutes. Be sure to pace yourself to allow enough time to play all three dogs' visits to the vet while still leaving around ten minutes for the final story/activity below.

Activity 3: Vet visit, reversed roles

Now, you will transition to another vet visit, but this time, you will reverse roles with the child, where you place the child in charge of controlling the vet, and you take on the role of playing the anxious animals. This role reversal gives the child a chance to demonstrate their retention of what they've learned in therapy so far and helps build additional mastery by having them "teach" their skills to someone else (in this case, to the bird(s) in this story).

To make the transition, close the last activity by having the vet say goodbye appropriately to the dogs (and if their illness seems to require a check-up later, perhaps the vet can set another appointment with them). At the end, have the vet say, "Now I need to go check on some bird friends of mine. I have to drive to go see them."

Then, get the jeep and the three wild birds (two parrots + toucan). Place the three birds on their perches and set them across the table or room. Then, have the vet load the jeep with any supplies that will fit and drive to see the birds. The description in this scene uses very specific toys that not all therapists may have in their current set. If possible, new therapists may wish to shop in advance of this session to find toys that will fit the needs of the session. Alternatively, you are welcome to browse your current selection and find suitable replacements. To fit the context of this scene, you only need three animals of similar species, with one that has a noticeable difference from the others. In this example, a toucan and two parrots are used. The toucan is depicted as having (catastrophic) anxiety about something being wrong with its beak. It doesn't understand why it looks different from the other birds, and thinks that something must be very wrong. So, any combination of animals that can fit a similar context can work: two horses and a giraffe, two pigs and a hippo, two cows and a goat, etc. Any variation of the classic "ugly duckling" story can work (see Figure 8.4).

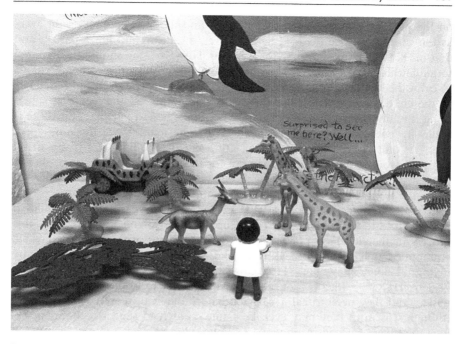

Fig. 8.4 This image shows a variation on activity 5.3. In this case, rather than birds, the vet visits with two giraffes and a gazelle. Photo by author

Set up the scene as follows:
[Key: R = red bird, B = blue bird, T = toucan, N = Narrator]

N: The vet is driving to go visit the birds, but the birds are very far away, so it takes him a while to get there. Meanwhile, the birds are talking to each other.

R (TO T): Hey, did you ever ask a doctor to look at your beak for you?

T: Not yet. I don't know why it is so much bigger than yours, but it's really freaking me out, man!

B: Yeah, dude, that thing is HUGE! I hope that doctor gets here soon before something bad happens!

T: Like what?

R: I don't know, man, but that can't be good! That's the most crazy, big beak I've ever seen on a parrot.

N: The vet is here now. [To child] You be the vet, and I'll be the birds. How does the story end?

Hopefully, the child will attempt to resolve the problem with only minimal guidance from you. In fact, experience has shown that most children pick up on the premise of this story rather quickly, and they work almost right away as the vet to convince the bird he is, in fact, a toucan, and not a parrot, and that his beak is supposed to be the way it is. However, you should be prepared to guide the play as necessary to assist the child in making recommendations to calm the birds. Playing as the birds, you should apply some mild resistance to the child's attempts to calm the birds, elaborating on the fear that something is really wrong with the toucan (who thinks he is a parrot). This scene is meant to evoke a sense of irrationality to some fears. Since the only "problem" is that the toucan is a toucan, not a parrot, the birds are really afraid for no reason. If this theme is apparent for the child, your goal, then, should be to help the child identify that irrationality. If the child does not identify the irrationality, you may consider leading them toward that conclusion.

Overall, your most important role in this reversal is to force the child to work a little to calm your own catastrophic anxiety. You want to make this process neither too easy nor too hard for them. Thus, if they try to convince you immediately that your beak is normal, you can put up some resistance by saying, "I don't know," or, "How can I believe you? I mean, *look* at me! My beak is HUGE!" Ideally, you can put up enough resistance to get them to understand they need to calm you first before they can reason with you, and (though it is rare) they may even be astute enough to suggest calming activities they have learned in previous sessions (i.e., relaxation stories or muscle relaxation). If not, you can pull away from the scene momentarily as needed to suggest to the child to try helping the bird relax first so that he will be less panicked and more able to listen. Then, you can proceed as needed with the child coaching you (the bird) how to relax, and you can follow their directions, whatever those may be (even if they seem a bit "non-traditional"). Once they begin coaching you in relaxation techniques, it is wise to pull up any resistance and go along with the relaxation smoothly, especially in this first "walkthrough" of the child playing "therapist." You do not want to frustrate the child by making it overly difficult to calm. Instead, you want to put up enough resistance only to push them to realize they need to calm you first, then you can calm rather quickly once they make that transition. Once calm, you can then receive the message that your beak is perfectly normal.

To close this activity and session as a whole, review with the child the underlying meaning of the activity (fighting catastrophic thinking). Start by reviewing the story and normalizing that feeling. After the story is completed, you may say, "You see, a lot of birds and people have the problem where they worried or get nervous because they think something is really bad when it's really not bad at all. Once they figure out it's not so bad though, they don't have to worry anymore and can finally just go on and live their lives. But sometimes, they need someone to help them realize it's not so bad." You may even consider giving them a "homework" assignment to look for times this week they engage in catastrophic thinking themselves and encourage them to use the techniques practiced today to help relax their worries.

Session 6

Purpose

Review previously learned material. To gauge child's perception of progress so far. To encourage self-evaluation and self-reward in the child. To solidify/further practice skill acquisition.

Goals

1 Review physiology and relaxation
2 Review anxious cognitions and coping strategies
3 Assess child's evaluation of what they have learned and whether they have practiced outside of therapy
4 Stimulate self-reward
5 Practice material presented previously

Session 6 begins the "practice" phase of FELT, in which you are no longer focused heavily on introducing new concepts or new skills, but, rather, using play to help build confidence and achieve mastery of skills learned so far. By this session, you should have a fairly strong case conceptualization for your client, and you should be able to identify and outline a majority of the essential features included in the FELT etiological model as described in Chapters 6 and 7.

So far, in overarching session goals, we have focused mainly on *manifest* factors in our anxious model. Consideration of *propagating* factors has occurred, and you've likely responded to some propagating factors already in earlier sessions, but a major focus of treatment was still on manifest factors. Now, however, we shift our interest more emphatically and explicitly toward propagating factors, and, similarly, formulate a plan for addressing them in future sessions. By now, you will have had an ample supply of play for analysis, which can help you draw meaningful hypotheses about potential psychodynamic factors influencing your client's anxiety. It is essential at this stage to take a moment to collect your thoughts about sessions so far and look for recurring themes within the FELT model of play analysis. A child who has had repeated instances of *deus ex machina* resolutions, for example, would likely need a plan to rehearse and execute more generalizable, realistic coping skills to add to their repertoire. A child who has constantly depicted an inept or ineffective Self in play would need intervention focused on building confidence and self-efficacy. As referenced in the conceptualization example given previously, you should also create plans to identify and address psychological needs that have arisen in play. For example, if your analysis reveals a child has shown recurring themes of unmet analgesia needs, you may consider creating stories for future sessions that force the child to manage times they cannot escape from pain, but, rather, must focus on soothing skills. Similarly, you may note that a child's previous play showed numerous themes of feeling "out of control," or like they have no sense of authority in their world. This would translate to hypotheses that the child may need to address *exousia* needs, and you would start to make a plan to consider play interventions where you can help the child address a need to feel *exousia*-like power, and that they have choices and authority in their world.

You should also create a plan as needed for other propagating factors. Starting in session 7 and especially in sessions 8–12, you will focus almost exclusively on "targeted" story stems – ones you create/adapt for your specific client to fit their specific needs. So, you will need to be armed with a good formulation to guide the creation of these stories. Though this session (session 6) does not include targeted stems, it is designed partially as a review for you as therapist to see what the child has retained regarding coping skills and needs, so you can properly plan ahead for ongoing sessions. Your formulation will influence what areas you may wish to emphasize in activity 3.

Activity 1: Physiology and relaxation

Invite the child to repeat physiology and relaxation activity as performed in previous sessions.

Activity 2: Anxious thoughts review

Use the following story stem to work with the child on anxious thoughts, as described in session 5.

Story: Missing baby elephant

Toys needed: elephant mother, elephant baby, African predators (e.g., lion, tiger, alligator, snake), friendly African animals (e.g., rhino, zebra, gorilla, friendly lion, etc.), trees, watering hole (a blue cloth, paper, or anything else that can represent water).

Set up the scene such that several friendly animals are gathering around the watering hole for a drink and/or bath. Feel free to use whatever animals you like, just as long as several are placed. Away from this scene, set up some trees, boulders, and/or another "blockade" (something an animal can hide behind) and place some predators behind the blockade. The predators should be placed within a relatively short "roaming" distance, as in this story, the baby elephant will roam away from its mother, risking being caught by the predators. However, they should not be placed so close that one might expect all the animals at the watering hole to realize their presence. If you are limited on space, you can simply instruct the child to imagine the distance is great enough so that the baby elephant essentially gets "lost" and cannot quickly or easily find the way back to the watering hole. As you are setting the scene, begin the story as follows:

> "One very hot day, all the animals were gathering around this watering hole where they could drink some water or get in the water to cool down. There was a ____, and a ____, and a _____ [you should name each of the animals present as you place them]. The mama elephant is getting water in her trunk and spraying it all over herself to cool off, while the baby plays in the water nearby. Then, while the mama is spraying herself, the baby gets out of the water and decides to go explore. The baby wandered off [baby elephant should walk toward the hidden predators at this point] and before she knew it, she was lost! [Here, you leave the baby near the predators, but you do not specify whether the predators or the baby realize each other is there.] Then, the mama realized the baby was gone, and she started to get worried! How does the story end?"

In this story, there are several characters who might show anxiety. You already stated within the story that the mother elephant was worried; however, the baby elephant could become worried as well (especially if separation anxiety is an issue for your child client). Furthermore, some of the friendly animals around the watering hole could share in the worry.

Likewise, there are several possible "helpers" in this story. The friendly animals may assist in calming the mother, trying to help reassure her and offering emotional support. They may also provide instrumental assistance and could help find the baby for the mother.

There are also several expectable ways for the story to end. The mother could find the baby immediately. The baby could hide playfully behind the tree, waiting to jump out and "scare" the mother. The baby could also wander even closer to the predators and put itself in danger. It was common in our studies for some children to even "ignore" the danger of the predators and to make the predator animals friendly as well, watching over baby or even helping the baby elephant back home. Whatever the case, your task in this story will be to help the child explore any anxiety present in any of the characters, and guide the child toward the identification of any potential anxious thoughts, feelings, and/or sensations. You should also use characters in the play as much as necessary to guide the child toward healthy coping skills in response to demonstrated anxiety. Interventions should take a form similar to those explained previously within this manual.

Timing for this activity should be around 15 minutes to leave enough time for activity 3, which is the main focus of this session.

Activity 3: Assessment and reward

This activity is designed to stimulate the child to assess responses to anxiety and reward demonstrations of positive coping skills as necessary. To that end, guidance and suggestions you offer as therapist should attempt to lead the child to identify healthy and maladaptive coping skills and to reward any efforts toward positive coping.

Part 1: Self-efficacy – the mountain of worry

The first part of this activity is meant to evoke a sense of self-efficacy in the child. This is done to "prime" the child toward identifying personal strengths. In this part, the child is asked to identify characteristics of the Self that are good using toys as representations of those characteristics. The scene invites the child to accomplish a presumably difficult task and identify strengths as they go about accomplishing that task.

In this activity, you will draw a mountain on a large piece of paper or flattened box for the child to climb using their Self-toy. Stacked blocks are used as scaffolding to climb the mountain. The mountain is labeled with various things the child worries about, and the blocks are labeled with healthy coping skills or other positive attributes the child uses to face difficult tasks. In treatment development, therapists used poster board or flattened cardboard boxes on which to draw the mountain, depending on what was available. The paper/box should be large enough that you can draw a mountain that spans about 24 inches (61 cm) at the base and is 24 inches (61 cm) tall at the apex. These are "rough" measurements though. The height of your mountain should ideally be measured to specifically fit the height of four stacked boxes/blocks, as described below, and thus will vary depending on the height of each box/block you choose.

In treatment development, empty cereal boxes were used for the stacking boxes. For uniformity, I wrapped them in plain black wrapping paper, but, interestingly, the wrapped boxes led some children to believe that these boxes were gifts to be unwrapped, leading some to be (mildly) disappointed when they discovered it was just an empty box. Since then, I no longer wrap the boxes, and kids do not seem to mind. Currently, my clinical practice is situated in a pediatric primary care office, and I use boxes in which samples of formula and baby food were shipped, as each of these is about 5 inches (12 cm) tall, and thus a good size for my 22-inch (56-cm) mountain (which is drawn on a flattened box). The boxes should have different dimensions though, to allow stepwise stacking. So, the base-layer block will be the widest and the top block the narrowest. For the mountain, I have found with experience that a flattened box works better than poster board because it can be made into an L-shape and stood against the wall, without falling over. When using poster board, we commonly had to tape it to the wall, which took up unnecessary time in session and risked (minor) damage to the wall if removed. Lastly, you will also need to size the mountain and blocks based on what you expect the child's "Self-toy" selection to be. By now, you should have a good idea about what toys your client seems most drawn to, and thus should know which ones may likely be their Self-toy. If there are Self-toy candidates that are rather tall, you may consider drawing a taller mountain for a more realistic feel to the activity. A 12-inch-tall Barbie doll, for example, would not be expected to have much trouble with an 18-inch mountain, but a 2-inch Lego figure would find the mountain appropriately enormous.

Toys needed: large piece of paper, such as poster board. A flattened cardboard box may also be used. Child's "Self-toy," stackable blocks, sticky notes, marker.

(This activity was adapted from a strategy suggested in Crenshaw, 2006.)

Tell the child that the mountain is the "Mountain of Worry" and have the child label the mountain with several worries. Usually, the child simply states different worries, while the therapist writes them on sticky notes in marker (using a marker, instead of a pen or pencil, allows for larger font, which is easier to read from distance). Then the therapist gives the notes to the child to post onto the mountain. Often, children use the mountain to create a hierarchy of anxiety, with less significant fears/worries at the bottom and more bothersome ones at the top. After labeling worries, you then go back to each worry and label them with thoughts/symptoms that arise when faced with the worry. These are then pasted next to or under the worries. Again, you should collaborate with the child to identify these, and you can help focus their descriptions as needed for accuracy.

After labeling the Mountain of Worry, the child will then "climb" the mountain by stacking blocks from the base toward the top. With each block, the child should name a coping skill, strength, or other good quality, which will be written on a sticky note and taped to the block. Frequently, children do aim to name at least one coping skill learned in previous sessions of FELT, but if they do not do so independently, you can suggest they add those skills as well. It is actually rather common to suggest at least one or two skills/strengths to add. Generally, you will stack four blocks to climb, but children usually identify five to six strengths/coping skills. So, some blocks may be labeled with multiple strengths/skills. As each block is labeled, it is placed atop another (or at the bottom of the mountain, if the first block), and the child places their Self-toy on top of the block. The idea is that the child will "stand on" their strengths to overcome the climb to the top of the mountain.

As therapist, you should explicitly note to the child that the only way to conquer/"climb over" the whole mountain of worry was to use several blocks/skills and combine them together. Although some worries (i.e., those at the bottom of the mountain) could be conquered with only a few blocks, all of them were needed to overcome the entire mountain. Your goal is to make it clear to the child that sometimes they may need to use an array of combined skills/supports to successfully master their anxiety fully.

At the end of the activity (when the child has reached the top of the mountain), you may congratulate the child on their climb or provide some other verbal reward. Also, collect the notes used to label the mountain and allow the child to keep them. You should stick them together in a sort of "booklet" form and then give this to the child (actually, in most cases, I give this to the parent when reviewing the session with them briefly at the end). Children and parents are typically instructed that the notes can be reviewed at home as a way to remember how strong they are and that they can "conquer really tough things" with the right supports. I have also encouraged parents to plan an activity at home where they turn the notes into a more durable "book," or some other creative activity, with their child. This not only promotes retention as a homework assignment between sessions, but it helps the parent become more directly engaged in understanding what skills/strengths the child is learning for managing anxiety.

[OPTIONAL, if time allows] Part 2: Encouragement and self-assessment

It is unusual for much or any session time to remain for Part 2 of this activity, but if you do find yourself with an extra ten minutes or so this session, you may proceed with the following activity, which continues to solidify the goal of building self-efficacy.

> "In this activity, you used things that you are good at to accomplish something hard. You had to think about yourself and figure out what you are good at so those could be your blocks to stand on. Now, I want to see if you can help someone else do something hard by kind of doing the same thing. Do you remember a long time ago you made up a story to show me what 'scared' or 'worried' was like? Now we're going to do that again. Do you want to make up a new one or use one you have done before?"

[If the child wants to use a previous scene, you may help by describing the story as necessary to help the child remember. You may reference any story created by the child in which a character exhibited anxiety. Usually, earlier examples are better, because such examples are expected to represent more maladaptive responses to anxiety, as they occurred before the child began to learn healthier coping responses. A good reference point may be the story created in session 2, activity 3. Nonetheless, any prototype may be used here.]

Whatever story the child chooses or creates, you should facilitate its development as much as necessary, continuing to use the overarching principles of FELT as in other sessions. This time, however, at appropriate points within the story, you should invite the child to come up with ways that the anxious character can address his/her anxiety. You, may, for example, say, "I wonder what _____ should do about being worried in this story?" If necessary, you may press further, "Do you remember what has worked for you so far to help when you start to have/think [insert appropriate symptom, e.g., 'butterflies in the stomach,' or thought, e.g., 'Oh no, I'm going to mess everything up']?" Your primary concern here should be to elicit the child to demonstrate what they have learned. You should then invite the child to reward themself for displaying their skills (e.g., "Do you think _____ did a good job in this story?" or, "Do you think ____ feels any better?"). If the child answers no, you should invite discussion about why not and allow the child to construct ways to help ____ feel better. This discussion should help lead you, as therapist, to learn what areas the child may be still seeking aid in and what concepts may need to be reviewed more extensively in subsequent sessions. If there is no time in session 6 for this activity, it can be delayed and used instead in future sessions.

Session 7

This is a review session. In this session, you will review with the child all the coping skills developed in the previous six sessions. Most of the activities will resemble those performed in session 6. Intervention strategies should continue to mirror those utilized throughout FELT.

Before this session, be sure to speak with the child's parents about how she has used skills outside of therapy (at home, school, etc.). Try to find out about a specific incident that the parents remember, as that incident (if available) will be used in activity 3. If no such example is named, ask the parents about any times the child has struggled with anxiety recently. That example can still be of use in activity 3. Also, tell the parent(s) they may be invited to join you with their child at the end of the session.

Purpose

To review all previously learned material in preparation for the prolonged practice stage.[5] To continue to strengthen the child's ability to cope with anxiety.

Goals

1) Review previous skills, including physiology and relaxation, changing anxious thoughts, and recognizing and rewarding the Self for a job well done.
2) Determine what skills, if any, the child tends to struggle with more, so that you may focus on strengthening those skills in remaining sessions.

Activity 1: Physiology and relaxation

Repeat as before.

Activity 2: Anxious thoughts

Use the following stem to review anxious thoughts (as in previous sessions).

Stem: Music concert

Toys needed: four children with musical instruments; additional people toys for the audience.

Similarly to the Vet stem in session 5, this session will set up multiple characters with differing levels of anxiety. In contrast to the Vet stem, though, this time a fourth character is added – someone who is "very nervous, but who has had help from a therapist and knows how to deal with their worries." By adding this fourth character, you are giving the child an opportunity to

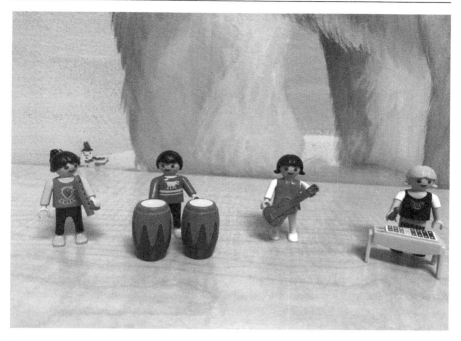

Fig. 8.5 A basic set-up for the Music concert stem, close up, no audience. Photo by author.

Self-identify with that toy and then to use their skills to potentially help others, thus increasing mastery. To create the scene, set up the children on (an imaginary) stage, each holding a different musical instrument. Each child will be "assigned" a different level of confidence. One child should feel confident about his/her skill. Another should be "only a little nervous, but thinks they can get by okay." One child should be "very nervous," and the last should be "very nervous like the other one, but has had help (from a therapist) and knows how to deal with their worried feelings." You should pair with your client to decide which toy gets assigned which role.

Next, set up a large audience to watch the concert – the larger the better, but try not to get carried away and spend too much time setting up hundreds of toys in the audience. Next, introduce the story stem as follows:

> "These children are getting ready to put on a concert for the school and families. [If necessary, relabel the children according to level of nervousness.] The curtain is closed right now, and they are backstage getting ready. [Review each one and have the child describe what each is feeling and thinking.] The teacher comes and tells them the curtain will open in five minutes and they should do whatever they need now to get ready. What happens next?"

Now, play turns over to the child, who explains each character's experience (as done in previous sessions). As before, you should invite the child to elaborate on each experience such that the child is able to explore the different components of the various levels of anxiety. This time, you may also add an evaluative component, where the "child who has had help" also comments on good things the other children are doing or helps the child(ren) who is/are struggling. Ideally, through the play, the child progresses through the concert and completes the stem. Some children may work to relax each child and then end right as the curtain opens. If this occurs, you should work to prolong the story a bit by having the child continue to talk about how the characters manage their feelings during the concert too. As usual in FELT, work to help direct the story to a healthy resolution.

Activity 3: Self-efficacy review

Invite the child to use the toys to show you a time during the past week (or any other time) that they have used the skills learned in therapy to help themself. If they cannot think of one, use the example given by their parents. If a positive example is not available from home, school, etc., focus on examples from past therapy sessions. A previously used scene may even be repeated, if necessary (as described in activity 6.3.2). If no positive examples can be found in any environment, you may choose the example given by the parents of a time the child struggled with anxiety. You can then ask the child to use the toys to show you the scene and what they would do differently.

Sessions 8–12+

These sessions are lumped together as "practice" sessions. For the remainder of therapy, your goal as therapist is to invite the child to practice their skills in as many different environments and scenarios as possible and necessary. Use the creative nature of play to design several symbolic representations of anxiety-ridden situations, and work with the child through play to practice healthy coping responses in those various situations. You should continue to invite the child to perform activities previously repeated (i.e., physiology and relaxation). Most of these sessions will greatly resemble session 7, though with different story stems and scenarios used. As much as possible, design story stems that target specific problem areas for your client. Key in this stage is that you will now be using your FELT case conceptualization more directly to plan and execute targeted story stems, designed to address remaining core issues. Chapter 11 is dedicated to describing how to formulate your own story stems.

Your goals throughout these sessions are as follows.

Goals

1 Practice previously learned skills including relaxation, changing anxious thoughts, and self-evaluation and reward.
2 Child moves toward and exhibits mastery of these skills.
3 Child demonstrates utilization of skills outside of therapy and/or demonstrates measurable decreases in anxiety outside of therapy.
4 Child moves toward healthy Object-relations and other psychological needs consistent with developmental expectations.

You should continue therapy to the extent necessary to achieve these goals. At the beginning of session 8, you should initiate this "prolonged practice" phase of FELT with a transition statement for the child similar to the following: *"In all the times we've met so far, we've learned a lot about anxiety, fears, worries, and nervousness. We've also used the toys and other games to learn how to deal with those feelings in a good, healthy way. Now, we're going to use those same skills to play through more examples of times someone might be scared, nervous, or worried. Like always, we'll help the toys and the characters so their problems don't feel too big to handle."* From there, you should check with the child that they understand, and then you will transition to your first story for session 8, which may be either a targeted stem you have prepared yourself, a revisiting of a former story that you feel will help address a core factor, or a story the child develops on their own during the session.

Below are listed a variety of potential story stems that may be used in this final stage as deemed appropriate by you and the child. Each story stem sets up potentially anxious scenarios for the child to complete. The child should be invited and allowed to practice resolving core issues remaining from their conceptualization. It is common at this stage for children to begin to show preferences for certain coping strategies, and it is okay to allow the child freedom to decide which copings skill(s) seem(s) more helpful for them (you don't need to "force" certain strategies). In some cases, stories may be completed such that the characters do not exhibit any anxious behaviors. When this occurs, you should emphasize what a good job characters did at healthily avoiding anxiety (i.e., you might say, "He never even started to worry because of....!"). You may also ask the child to "replay" any of the scenes, but with a different ending (i.e., "Now show me how it would go if ____ were to use some more of the skills we learned in here.").

It is generally advised that the story stem examples below be kept as "backups" should you need them in session to fill time (e.g., if the targeted stems you prepared for your client prove not to take as much time as you anticipated). Alternatively, you can use these sample stems to generate your own ideas and to adapt to create targeted stems for your client. Additional guidelines for creating your own story stems are included in Chapter 11.

You should also be aware that approximately two to three sessions before you plan to end therapy, you will also begin to discuss and prepare for termination/graduation from therapy. This process is outlined in Chapter 10, with some sample story stems relevant to termination offered.

Note: throughout these stories, characters are arbitrarily named for the sake of simplicity. In presenting the stories yourself, you may choose a different name, allow the child to name characters, or simply describe the characters by their generic name (i.e., the boy, the dog, etc.). Also, unless otherwise specified, the toys used may be set up in any logical manner that fits the story stem.

Story stems

Going to the doctor

(Good for medical anxiety or general nervousness about the unknown.)

Toys needed: clinic, doctor, child, parents, medical supplies, table.

Introduction: "Jimmy has been feeling really sick for a few days. His head hurts very badly. His parents decided to take him to the doctor for a checkup. Jimmy and his parents went into the doctor's office and the doctor told him to sit on the table. Jimmy was pretty nervous because he thought something was really wrong with him. He had all kinds of nervous feelings and thoughts and didn't know what to do with them. What happens next?"

Parental quarrel

(Good for anxiety about adult concepts.)

Toys needed: parents, furniture, two children.

Introduction: "Molly and her friend Grace were playing in Molly's room at Molly's house. Grace had come over today after school. Molly's parents were in the other room. Molly and Grace were playing with their dolls when they heard Molly's parents start to argue. They heard Molly's mom yell, 'I can't believe you did that!' Molly's parents don't usually argue. They are usually very happy and love each other very much. Molly didn't know what to do. She started thinking to herself. Now show me what she was thinking, and what happens next?"

The speed test

(Good for test- or other performance-related anxiety.)

Toys needed: lion, tiger, bear, zebra.

Introduction: "The lion, tiger, bear, and zebra were walking home from school together. They were all talking about a big test they had tomorrow. It was called the 'Speed test,' and it was a really important test because they all had to pass it to go on to the next grade. To pass the test, you had to be able to run 30 mph. The lion, tiger, and zebra were all talking about how they would pass the test easily. The lion said, 'I can run 50 mph, so I'll beat that by a long shot!' The tiger said, 'I can run 45, so I'll be fine too.' The zebra said, 'I can only run 40, but that's definitely enough to pass.' The bear was quiet. He knew the fastest he had ever run was 30 mph, and that was only one time! He wasn't sure if he could do it again.

"What happens next?"

Stealing

(Good for anxiety about doing the right thing, social anxiety, and anxiety about bullying.)

Toys needed: bear, bunny, safari man, tent, computer, "general goods" (flowers, food, supplies – anything that could be sold to animals in a general store).

Safari man should be standing under the tent, facing toward outside. The computer should be just in front of him. It should resemble a kiosk, with the computer functioning as a "checkout." Place some goods around the kiosk.

Introduction: "Bob has a store where he sells _____ [list things]. He has two shoppers in his store today: a bunny and a bear. Bob was looking down on his computer while the animals shopped. The bunny was smelling some flowers when he saw the bear take (something relatively valuable) and put it in his pocket. The bunny looked at Bob to see if he was watching, but Bob wasn't. He didn't see anything. The bunny knew that it was wrong for the bear to steal, but the bunny was afraid that if he told, the bear would get mad and eat him. He wanted to do the right thing, but he was scared.

"What happens next?"

The sleepover

(Good for separation anxiety and anxiety about trying new things.)

Toys needed: children; a parent, set of parents, or guardian(s); any other sleepover supplies as needed.

Introduction: "Violetta is attending her first ever sleepover. She is going to a friend's house, along with three other friends from school. Violetta has never slept at someone else's house before, and she is pretty nervous about being away from home. She really wants to stay the whole night though, so she doesn't miss out on any fun. The sleepover already started, and Violetta is there at the house. The girls have all been having a good time, but it's starting to get dark outside, and Violetta knows it will be bedtime soon. She starts to feel nervous. What happens next?"

Illness anxiety and anxiety about starting a new school

(Good for general contamination anxiety and/or for anxiety about starting something new and unfamiliar.)

Introduction: "Diego is a third grader who has been homeschooled for several years now, since the beginning of COVID. His mother has a problem in her lungs that would make it very serious for her if she got COVID, so Diego's family has been very careful from the start to follow all the right guidelines to keep everyone healthy. However, Diego and his family decided it was finally time for him to go back to traditional school for this new third-grade year. Diego is very nervous about going, though, because he hasn't been to a school in more than two years, and he doesn't know what to expect. He is also worried because he doesn't want to get his mother sick! His parents knew it would be hard for him and they got him some help from a counselor before going back to school. He's been in counseling for a couple months now, and it has helped him, but he is still feeling very nervous. Diego is at home and has just awoken on the morning he is supposed to start school. What happens next?"

Broken tablet

(Good for anxiety about getting in trouble or doing the wrong thing; also a good story to ask the child to "replay" to ask them to have Aleks do something different to prevent breaking the tablet in the first place.)

Introduction: "Aleks was playing a game in his room on his tablet. He had been playing for a while, and his mom told him it was time to get off. He was in the middle of a tough game, though, and wanted to finish before he quit. His mom said he could have five more minutes. Those five minutes passed, and he still wasn't finished. This time, his dad came in and told him, 'Alexs! It's time to get off.' Aleks still wasn't ready and asked for a few more minutes. Aleks' dad told him, 'No!' that it was time for dinner and he needed to get off. Aleks begged for one more minute, and Dad said, 'Fine, but you better be done when I come back.' Aleks' dad left for five more minutes before he came back. The dad gave Aleks extra time just in case, but Aleks still wasn't done. Dad saw Aleks still playing and got mad. 'Aleks! Turn it off now. You've had ten minutes!' Aleks started to feel angry because he didn't get to finish his game, and he didn't want to turn it off. Dad came to take the tablet away, but Aleks jerked away hard. He jerked away so hard that he lost control of the tablet and dropped it on the floor. Dad went to check and the screen was cracked. He yelled at Aleks and told him, 'That's it! You're grounded from the tablet and you're going to have to do double chores for a month to pay for the damage to the screen!' Aleks was surprised he broke the screen and felt guilty at first, but then when Dad started to yell he got scared. Except Aleks didn't act scared. Instead, he started to feel even more angry. What happens next?"

Late hate

(Good for children who stress about being late to places or who do not do well with changes in routine.)

Introduction: "Willow hates being late. Her teachers told her that if she is late to school more than five times in a year, her parents would have to do detention, and she wouldn't be allowed to participate in the attendance party for all the kids with perfect attendance. So, every morning before school, Willow got up really early and stressed out about being late. Meanwhile, Willow's brother didn't care at all about being late. He took forever to get ready every morning, and mom and Willow were always rushing him to get in the car. All this really stressed Willow out. One morning, Willow was already up and ready to leave, but her brother was still in the shower even though they needed to leave in five minutes. Willow had never been late before, but she was definitely going to be late this time. There was no way they would leave on time. Willow started to cry. What happens next?"

Defective detective

(Good for test/performance anxiety. Also good for anxiety about being different and for working on Self-identity in comparison to others. This story uses animals, instead of people, but people toys can easily be swapped in as desired.)

Introduction: "Detective Frank was the only turtle on the police force. You might be surprised to see a turtle policeman, especially when all the other police are big, strong, and fast animals. [Here you can list the other animals that you choose and that fit the description – lions, bears, bulls, cheetahs, etc.] All the other police animals made fun of Detective Frank because he was so slow. They would run past him every day in slow motion when they came in the office and would laugh about the time he tried to catch the bad guy, a hare/rabbit, but he couldn't keep up. One of them would pretend to be the hare/rabbit and speed off, while another one would run in slow motion while saying, 'Look at me! I'm Frank, and I'll never catch a bad guy!'

"Captain Stacy was Frank's new boss. She had come in from another town and taken over for Frank's former boss, his friend Chuck. Captain Stacy was testing all the detectives to find out who she wanted to keep and who she would fire. This made Frank really nervous. His test was scheduled for three days from now. What happens next?"

Child-specific stories

You should prepare at least one child-specific story stem for each session. You should create some situations that would be expected to evoke low-anxiety in the child, and some that would evoke high-anxiety. These should progress in frequency and intensity over time and as the child reaches skill mastery. The closer the child gets to the end of treatment, the more often that targeted, child-specific stories should be used.

Also, you can invite the child to create stories of their own and respond accordingly.

Repeated or unused stories

Finally, you may feel free to repeat stories used in previous sessions or use any that were listed, but unused in previous sessions. You may also create stems from some of the examples given in this manual.

Notes

1 In this table, "gendered" terms are used to refer to toys that represent the traditional "binary" definition of gender. These gendered terms refer to the representation of each toy's "expressed" gender, that is, the gender that the toy "shows" to the outside world. The terms have nothing to do with gender identity, and toys, by nature, have no specific identity. Instead, they allow children to project parts of themselves or others onto the toy. Thus, toys with "binary" genders can be used by children to represent non-binary states (a "male" toy can be called a "girl" if so desired, or vice versa). Similarly, the toys do not need to have any identified gender at all. It is best to follow the child's lead here, and therapists are encouraged to practice cultural competence in relating to children about "gendered" toys and "gendered" terms in the practice of psychotherapy.

2 In this manual, activities can be abbreviated by session and activity number. In this case, 2.3 means "session 2, activity 3."

3 Heart rate is simple to manipulate and to measure. This is why exercise or other physical activity is the primary suggested interoceptive exposure activity for this session, because it teaches the concepts clearly and simply. Thus, it is advised to select heart rate-increasing exposures often during the first few iterations of this activity, unless such exposures are contraindicated for the particular child being treated. If, for example, the child is unable to exercise due to a physical handicap, other methods and measurement techniques can be used as needed.

4 Horizontal refers to a relational hierarchy, Others he sees as roughly on the same level as the Self. Vertical relationships would signify those where Steve is either lower (as in with parents) or higher (as in with a much younger sister) on the hierarchy.

5 In reality, the child has been practicing skills throughout FELT. However, after the final review conducted here in session 7, the child will enter a stage in which new skills are no longer introduced and no more "generalized" story stems are used, but the child is allowed multiple opportunities to practice those skills for the remainder of therapy with "targeted" stems only. This is what is meant by "prolonged" practice.

REFERENCE

Crenshaw, D. (2006). *Evocative Strategies in Child and Adolescent Psychotherapy.* Lanham, MD: Jason Aronson.

Chapter 9

Parent component

Studies have shown the addition of a parent component to significantly increase the effect of psychotherapy on children (Bratton et al., 2005). Parental involvement in FELT is meant to help improve the child's overall response to therapy by utilizing the inherent closeness of the parent–child relationship to facilitate the child's overall sense of security and to increase generalization of skills outside the "therapy room." As a result, parents' involvement in FELT takes place both at home and within actual sessions between the child and therapist. The therapist helps the parents learn skills they may teach their child when anxiety-provoking stimuli inevitably arrive so that they may help the child when the therapist cannot be present. The therapist also helps the parents foster a sense of security in their own ability to help the child when struggling with anxiety (and other high emotionality). Parents learn how to encourage and facilitate their child's fantasy play so that its potential therapeutic benefits are maximized.

In this chapter, a parent-only session is described relatively loosely, to allow individualization of the session as needed. Therapists using this book are expected to already have some general knowledge about managing a parent-only session, and so I do not devote as much space here to reviewing general principles of working with parents in psychotherapy. Rather, the description below contains primary goals and tasks of the parent-only session, and therapists are allowed some discretion in how they communicate those goals to parents. Following that description is a portrayal of how parents are expected to interact with children during a joint session and during "homework."

Parent-only session (in development studies, this came after session 3 with child)

Purpose

To encourage parental cooperation in the treatment program.

DOI: 10.4324/9781032693187-11

Goals and tasks

1   To provide additional information about the treatment. Outline the treatment program and explain generally where the child is in treatment and what will happen next (a movement toward learning, and mastering, specific skills to manage anxiety). Invite and answer questions from parents. Remind parents not to expect an immediate reduction in anxiety, but that over time, changes should occur.

2   To give parents an opportunity to discuss concerns about the child or other factors that could influence treatment. Use open-ended questions to invite additional history or current information that may be pertinent to treatment or to understanding the child.

   a   **"How do you feel things have gone so far? Have you noticed additional concerns in your child that have come up since we started? Were there other things that have come to mind that you haven't mentioned that you feel I should know about?"**

3   To learn more about specific anxiety-provoking situations for the child and their specific reactions to such events. Use information garnered from initial sessions to discuss general impressions so far and to inform the discussion about client-specific anxiety. Parents are encouraged to provide their own impressions as desired.

   a   **"Tell me about a time recently that you've noticed your child was anxious? What triggered the reaction and what was their reaction? How did you feel when you noticed they were anxious?"**

   b   **"As I've gotten to know your child in therapy, I've noticed a few things about their anxiety that I wanted to discuss.** [The following is an example to illustrate a possible line of questioning.] **First, I've noticed that in anxious situations during play, your child seems repeatedly worried they will get in trouble for doing something wrong. Now this isn't an uncommon worry in young children, and it doesn't necessarily mean you're doing anything wrong as parents. Kids just don't like to get in trouble. But, I'm curious if you notice things like that at home. Do you notice times when your child seems to avoid telling you something because they're afraid you'll be angry?"**

4   To outline how parents may be involved in the program. Parents are advised that they will be invited to sit in on their child's next therapy session (session 4), so that they can witness the treatment model and learn useful interventions that they can implement with their child. Parents are informed that such participation is not mandatory, but are encouraged that doing so should be reasonably expected to greatly improve their child's response to therapy and is likely to facilitate

progress through the program. They are then encouraged to practice skills learned through their involvement with their child at home.

a   **"We're getting ready to enter the phase in therapy where you will get to be more involved as parents in learning what coping skills your child is learning and then how you can reinforce those at home. I'll be inviting you into the second half of the session the next time your child comes, so we can show you what we've done, and I'll also be showing you additional things along the way in other sessions that you can do at home with your child. We know from research that the more involved you can be at home, the more likely your child will retain coping skills and use them when they need them."**

5   To further interview parents about parenting styles in order to identify patterns that might be considered risk or protective factors with respect to their child's anxiety and to prepare parents to potentially make changes to their interactions with their children in order to stimulate their child's adherence to treatment recommendations. You should assess for features within the following realms:

a   Punitiveness (how do they respond when their child does something wrong?)

    i   **"How do each of you** [if child has only one parent, adapt language accordingly] **approach correcting your child when they do something wrong?"**

    ii   As therapist, you want to listen for cues of poor emotional control in parents, and then provide recommendations as needed to help them better model emotional stability with children.

b   Avoidance of affect (in general and specific to anxiety)

    i   **"Let's think about a time when you yourselves are experiencing a strong emotion. How do you tend to respond to those emotions? What about when someone else is emotional? How do you tend to respond to that?"**

c   Anxiety about their child's anxiety (vicarious anxiety)

    i   **"Now let's think about times when your child is anxious. How do you tend to feel when you notice your child is anxious? What if you're going to do something that you know might make them anxious, but they're not anxious yet? How do you tend to handle that?"**

d   Parental knowledge of healthy personal coping skills

    i   **"What are some ways you've found that work for you to cope with stress and other negative emotions? Even if you don't use them**

personally, what do you know about healthy ways other people might use to cope with strong emotions?"

ii   Philosophy about a parent's role in helping children with problems

iii   **"What is your parenting philosophy about how much or how often a parent should do something to help their child solve a problem or manage an emotion? Are there times you feel like it's better to 'sit back and watch,' and let them figure it out alone? What about the opposite? Are there times where you feel it's necessary to just 'take over' and do something for them? How do you work to find the right balance between encouraging independence versus providing help?"**

e   Willingness and ability to follow treatment recommendations

i   **"As we move forward in treatment, we'll be talking more and more about things you can do at home to help. Do you anticipate there being any barriers that might make it hard for you to participate in treatment?"**

f   Other specific factors that may have come up in play-themes with the child during initial sessions.

In response to these various questions with parents, you should, of course, provide intervention or recommendations as necessary to help inform parents about ways they can best support their child in a therapeutic manner. If issues come up that suggest a parent may benefit from their own psychotherapy, it can help to open up conversations about that as well. For example, "It sounds from our conversation like you, yourself, struggle with pretty significant anxiety too. Since you brought your child to see me, I can tell that it is important for you to help learn healthy ways to deal with anxious feelings. Have you ever had counseling yourself?" From there, you can help navigate the parent toward therapy of their own (with a different clinician) if that seems feasible or warranted.

Parents' involvement in session 4 with child and afterward

With the child's permission, parents are invited to observe and/or participate in a review of the "Physiology and relaxation" activity performed at the end of session 4. Parents may participate totally throughout each step (physiological activation, relaxation, and progressive muscle relaxation), or may simply listen/observe. Parents are particularly encouraged to play the "Righty Tighty, Lefty Loosey" game, as additional players may add to the fun, and their presence will allow them to be consistently reminded of the therapeutic purpose of the game.

Parents should also be continuously consulted about their child's progress and utilization of skills outside of therapy. Parental input can be very beneficial in assisting therapists' decision making about how and where to intervene. Parents should also be reminded often to note and reward their child's progress whenever possible. It is suggested that a formal, brief discussion with parents occur at least every four sessions (if not every session) for the purpose of evaluating the child's progress at home, identifying parental reactions to the therapy, and answering any lingering questions parents may have about how they can participate further in their child's treatment. Typically, such discussions can take place during the first five minutes of a regularly scheduled session with their child. Routine discussion with parents should also include some form of parent education about your case conceptualization – what you see as the core issues contributing to the child's anxiety and how you've noted that and then intervened through their play.

Preventing premature termination

A wealth of research on premature termination of psychotherapy with children has determined several major predictors of early termination. These predictors include avoidance behavior (Chasson, Vincent, & Harris, 2008) and parent factors, attitudes, and expectations such as less education, feeling that problems should be handled within the family, and using increased disciplinary tactics to respond to emotional/behavioral problems (McCabe, 2002). The latter-described factors can usually be easily identified and averted early in therapy by appropriately informing and educating parents about what they can expect from the treatment plan and involving them in at least some therapeutic interactions. Therefore, an essential part of the parent component of FELT is to ensure communication of a coherent, well-described treatment plan with parents so that the plan is clear and expectations are reasonable. The preliminary research on the FELT manual provides information about what kinds of behavioral changes parents can expect in their children and when they can expect those to occur. Communicating findings from previous research may help to alleviate uncertainties parents may have about what to expect from FELT. To review here, early FELT development research reviewed progress with parents every 4 weeks throughout the 12-week study (sessions were held once per week). At the end of week 4, approximately half of parents in the study commented they felt their child's anxiety had *worsened*. Qualitative reviews revealed this "worsening" was attributable to the fact that the first month of therapy focuses on enhancing expression of anxiety and emotion, which translated to children at home being more open and expressive about their worries/anxiety. Thus, in these cases, it became key to openly communicate with parents about this perceived worsening, to normalize it as a healthy response to therapy, and to reassure that anxiety will dissipate over time with consistent treatment. Eight-week reviews in the same study proved this to be true, with all parents who reported week 4 worsening describing improvement by week 8.

The other factor that predicts early termination, avoidance behavior, is a factor that is important to consider both for children *and* for their parents. Although the child may influence parents' decision to terminate, the parents do ultimately have the final decision to end or continue therapy. The current research has focused so far solely on avoidance behavior of the child (Chasson, Vincent, & Harris, 2008), and seems to indicate that when avoidance behavior begins to increase during therapy, anxiety also increases, and termination may begin being considered. Theoretically, though, avoidance behavior of the parent may be considered the true factor in the decision to terminate, since parents ultimately make the decision to consent or withdraw from treatment. The decision to terminate prematurely can be considered a manifestation of an avoidance of therapy. The parents may wish to avoid their anxiety about therapy itself (Hembree et al., 2003), or they may be avoiding the therapist (Chung, Pardeck, & Murphy, 1995). Parents themselves may feel vicarious anxiety about their child's anxiety about attending therapy (Chasson, Vincent, & Harris, 2008), which may lead them to terminate therapy prematurely. On the contrary, parents may display a different form of avoidance behavior. Some parents may prioritize their own anxiety about confrontation from the therapist over their inclination to terminate for their child's sake, and may "force" their children to persevere through therapy because they do not want to inconvenience the therapist by quitting. Regardless of the type of avoidance behavior occurring, one major purpose of regular parent contact by the FELT therapist is to reduce avoidance behavior by parents and to promote a healthy level of approach behavior instead. By encouraging parents to approach issues and/or concerns directly with the therapist, FELT clinicians can better target therapy to the entire context of their child clients. They can also respond appropriately to any parent factors that may be contributing to the propagation of anxiety in the child. Finally, they can help parents model approach behavior for their children, which, as stated previously, is a core feature in reducing anxiety.

Regardless of the complex influence of various factors related to anxiety about therapy, the point for FELT is that part of the therapist's job throughout FELT is to also help parents negotiate their own feelings about having their child in therapy. Doing so will not only facilitate therapist–parent interactions, but it will also reduce the likelihood that parents will remove their children from treatment before the child is ready. It will also maximize the parents' ability to participate in their child's therapy and to foster positive, healthy coping that the child is learning through therapy. Finally, by engaging in frequent interactions with parents (i.e., brief check-ins at the beginning and/or end of each session), FELT clinicians can better understand and direct therapy toward any parental factors that may be propagating anxiety in their children.

REFERENCES

Bratton, S. C., Ray, D., Rhine, T., & Jones, L. (2005). The efficacy of play therapy with children: a meta-analytic review of treatment outcomes. *Professional Psychology: Research and Practice*, 36(4), 376–390.

Chasson, G. S., Vincent, J. P., & Harris, G. E. (2008). The use of symptom severity measured just before termination to predict child treatment dropout. *Journal of Clinical Psychology*, 64(7), 891–904.

Chung, W. S., Pardeck, J. T., & Murphy, J. W. (1995). Factors associated with premature termination of psychotherapy by children. *Adolescence*, 30(119), 717–721.

Hembree, E. A., Foa, E. B., Dorfan, N. M., Street, G. P., Kowalski, J., & Tu, X. (2003). Do patients drop out prematurely from exposure therapy for PTSD? *Journal of Traumatic Stress*, 16(6), 555–562.

McCabe, K. M. (2002). Factors that predict premature termination among Mexican-American children in outpatient psychotherapy. *Journal of Child and Family Studies*, 11(3), 347–359.

Chapter 10

Termination

In this chapter, procedures for termination of FELT are described. Within this chapter, termination is defined as successful, planned termination that occurs as a result of a child having demonstrated a mastery of all skills learned during FELT such that symptoms of anxiety are no longer reported by the child or parent(s) as being unmanageable and/or clinical in nature. Under this definition, successful termination is never premature. Although procedures for premature termination may follow a similar format as those described below, this chapter's primary intention is to delineate a successful termination of psychotherapy. Within FELT, successful termination occurs when a child has met all goals of FELT as outlined in session guides, has demonstrated mastery over skills learned during FELT, and has reported a significant enough decrease in anxiety symptoms that the presenting problem is no longer described as an unmanageable issue that frequently interferes with daily functioning.

For most children, termination of psychotherapy can be an uncertain time in which several ambivalent feelings may be experienced. Although a child approaching successful termination may feel pride at having overcome anxiety and consequently may experience a readiness to move forward, that same child may simultaneously also feel a sense of sadness at the culmination of the therapeutic relationship that has been built between them and their therapist over the past 12+ weeks. Because of this ambivalence, termination of therapy requires the same amount of sensitivity and care as initial rapport-building during the initiation of therapy. At the same time, most school-aged children are accustomed to healthy, planned terminations of relationships with adult mentors, as they do so annually with teachers, coaches, etc. So, it is important for the therapist to recall that although the idea of termination can cause some mild stress on children and their families, it is usually a stress they have experienced and successfully managed before.

Termination marks a new era of uncertain expectations about the future. Children are likely to wonder, "Will I get worse or will I stay better?" "Will I ever see my therapist again?" "Will my therapist remember me?" and so on. Acknowledgement of ambivalence is an important step in beginning termination with children. Helping children navigate through the mysteries of these

DOI: 10.4324/9781032693187-12

ambivalent feelings is a key component of termination in FELT. With that consideration in mind, the following activities describe ways therapists work with children to prepare them for termination. I also describe in detail a final termination activity, reserved for the final planned session of FELT.

It is very important for clinicians to note that termination of psychotherapy does NOT occur in one session, but is rather better understood as a process that occurs over time. Termination actually begins with a preparatory stage two to three sessions before the actual final session in which children are informed of the impending end of therapy. Starting around two to three sessions prior to termination, FELT therapists commonly prepare a few *termination story stems*, which they work into the final sessions along with other targeted story stems. In FELT's 12-session treatment studies, these termination story stems began in session 10, during which children were advised they were reaching the end of therapy. The first step in successful termination is to create a celebratory nature to the idea of "graduating" from therapy. So, in telling children they are reaching the end of therapy, therapists work to use congratulatory and celebratory language, such as, "You've made it all the way to the end, and it's so exciting. I am very proud of you!" Celebratory language is usually how the conversation starts, but you should also make it clear that ambivalent feelings are normal. At that point, ambivalent feelings begin to be explored, discussed, and normalized. Therapists may, for example, express that "most kids feel kind of proud and relieved to have finally reached the end, but at the same time, kids usually don't really know what to think about how things might change now that they've gotten used to coming to therapy." Responses are elicited briefly from the child, and it is made clear that there will be time in the next several sessions to talk/play more about feelings about the end of therapy if the child wants to do so.

There a few common termination stems that therapists have used in FELT studies that have worked well. I will list these below for reference. Typically, therapists plan to use one termination stem per session in sessions 10 and 11, along with any other targeted stems they have planned to continue working on presenting problems.

Termination stems

A gorilla is released back into the wild

In this stem, you will create a zoo-like scene, focused on the gorilla exhibit of the zoo. At a minimum, you will need a gorilla toy, a cage/enclosure, and zookeepers. You and/or the child may wish to add other zoo animals to say "goodbye" to the gorilla, but this addition is not essential, as the focus in this scene is on the termination of the relationship between a caregiver (in this case, the therapist) and child, rather than among the child and their peers.

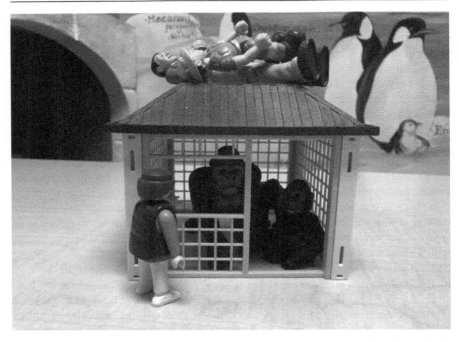

Fig. 10.1 Gorillas, after temporarily residing at the zoo, are preparing to be released back into the wild. In this image, some of the zoo staff slept on top of the enclosure to be near to the gorillas (an addition suggested by the child who played this scene). Photo by author.

You should set up the scene such that the gorilla is still in its enclosure, and you can select one or several zookeepers and place them around the enclosure. Next, introduce the scene as follows:

"A gorilla has been in the zoo for a while, but now the gorilla is getting ready to be released back into the wild. It has learned everything it needs to survive with the other gorillas in the wild, and tonight is its last night in the zoo. It will be released tomorrow morning. All the zookeepers in the zoo have gathered around to spend one last night with the gorilla. Tomorrow morning, the zookeeper closest to the gorilla will drive it out to the jungle to let it meet the other gorillas and join them. What happens next?"

Ideally, the child will take over play and start with reviewing what the zookeepers will do with the gorilla during that last night to say "goodbye." In FELT studies, children varied from relatively quick goodbyes, to giving hugs, to throwing a party, to having the zookeepers sleep next to or inside the enclosure all night. There is no real "healthy" prototype of a goodbye that you are trying to promote with the child, and the goal really is just to allow a proper goodbye of any kind and to generate positive, celebratory experiences.

So, should the child "skip" these goodbyes and move straight toward the gorilla's release, it can be helpful to direct the child to first start with "the night before" and play through those goodbyes with the zookeepers, even if they are relatively short. After these goodbyes, the child should then ideally move toward the gorilla's release, with you as therapist guiding them as needed toward a healthy resolution of the play stem, as you have done throughout FELT. Typically, children in FELT show little distress in play during this scene and rather intuitively "get" the celebratory nature of "graduation" from the zoo. However, you should be alert to any signs of distress and be prepared to respond accordingly and work through these emotions as needed.

A hospitalized child is released from hospital

This scene follows a similar idea as the gorilla scene, but this time uses a sick child who has gotten better and is being released from the hospital. The setup is nearly identical, where a child is spending their last night in the hospital and the treatment team (doctors, nurses, etc.) are saying goodbye. You do not need to name any certain illness that the child has and can just default to saying the child "was sick, but has gotten better and can go back home now." The scene typically plays out just as the gorilla scene does.

Other termination stories

You can also create/develop your own termination stories based on the interests of your particular client, following a similar trajectory/template as those referenced above. In all termination stories, it is advised to offer a realistic depiction of follow-up, depending on your setting. If it is possible the child may reasonably "see you around" in the future, it is okay to cast similar expectations in these play scenes. For example, you may mention that the zookeepers will "check in" on the gorilla every once in a while or that the doctors at the hospital are still available if the child ever needs them. If you do not expect to be able to offer such follow-up (perhaps you or the child are moving away to another state), you should be honest about this and offer other indicators of Object permanence. For example, "Even if they are not together, the gorilla and zookeepers will always remember each other, and the gorilla will remember what it learned in the zoo. So, even if things get scary out there in the jungle, the gorilla is ready and can think back on what they learned in the zoo for help whenever needed."

Termination session

This is the final session of FELT. It is the culmination of the work you did with the child and is scheduled as a celebration while also creating something together to enhance maintenance of therapeutic gains. You will work with the child to create a book that describes the most important things you did in therapy together. It will be a review of techniques and also a memory book of therapy as a whole. Starting two to three sessions before, you will have already told the child what to expect in this final session (that you will be creating a book together to take home). This way, the child is prepared for the "different" nature of this session, in that they will not be using toy-based play.

Termination activities

Goals

1   Promote permanence of therapy techniques
2   Promote Object permanence of therapist
3   Promote maintenance of gains
4   Promote continued practice and mastery of skills

Underlying each of these goals, again, is the desire of the therapist to help the child negotiate ambivalence about the end of therapy. Each goal is meant to alleviate worry about how things might change after therapy, thus driving internal attributions of the child to a state of "things will be alright, as they are now." Thus, the termination session as a whole is meant to celebrate gains, stimulate a sense of self-efficacy, and to share memories that the therapist has about time spent with the child. This latter component is a core feature that is meant to promote an internalization of the therapist Object. Theoretically, this therapist Object is hoped to accompany the child through life. Internalization means that children can use this "imaginary therapist" as a means to work through anxious situations as they grow into adulthood.

Activity: Termination book

The entire termination session is devoted to the co-creation of a termination book. Together, therapist and client construct a book that records memories from FELT. The book is about the child, and the title of the book always includes the child's name. The therapist prepares materials for the book before the final session. *Consequently, preparation for this session should begin several days before the scheduled session.* On average, it takes between one and two hours of prep time to create the necessary materials, excluding the time to print/develop photos for inclusion in the book (see below). A plain cover page introduces the book and contains the child's name, as well as any other creative title you wish to add, for example: *"Jason Jones, Fear Fighter Extraordinaire."* Inside, the book consists of photos or drawn pictures of scenes created during therapy, with a written narrative describing how each scene depicts the child and/or their progress across therapy. Each section of the book is described in more detail below.

Pre-session preparation

Before the termination session, the therapist must prepare all materials so that the actual time in the session can be spent reading through and constructing the book with the child. Preparation typically requires approximately one to two hours for each client, though the usage of templates often reduces this prep time considerably.[1] Additional time is necessary if photos are developed. The majority of prep time involves reconstructing some of the essential scenes used for the book. Planning and writing the actual narrative of the book also takes time. The book is written by the therapist, from the therapist's perspective, and tells about the child. The first step is to write a meaningful narrative of the child's experience in therapy, from start to finish. Examples are provided below. When writing the narrative, you will select relevant themes that seem important for the child to include in the book. Many of these may be generic stems, while others may be targeted. A guideline for the narrative is provided in Table 10.1 below.

Once you have written the narrative, you must now create a plan for the "artwork" of the book. In planning artwork, you must consider the time limitations you will have during your termination session (45–60 minutes). For this reason, it is not advised to allow the child to draw every scene, but you may wish to leave some drawing activities for the child, as many children do like to draw or decorate their book. I have found drawing and decorating the cover while using preprinted photos for the rest of the book to be a good use of time. You will be reading the book out loud with the child, one page at a time, while adding photos and decorations, and doing it this way can take up a fair amount of time. So, again, preprinted photos that the child pastes (with a glue stick) to the pages tends to be the most efficient way to add artwork. To create photos for printing, you will need to recreate scenes from your sessions with the child and take photos of the scenes. Your first time doing this takes the longest, but if you save photos, you will find that you can often use the same photos across multiple termination books, especially for generic stems that every child completes. Occasionally, scrupulous children may comment that your photo does not fit their memory of the scene perfectly, but this is okay and they are usually willing to forgive you while regaling you with a short story about how they remember it differently. This is a great opportunity to simply seek forgiveness for remembering it wrong and to reinforce with the child how they can use that great memory to their therapeutic advantage – "I'm so glad that you remember things so well. That will be great for you because it means you will always remember how to fight any other worries or anxieties that happen in the future."

Sample termination book

Actual FELT termination books are typically printed on 8.5 × 11 inch paper, using large (20+ point) font to improve readability for young children. This

Table 10.1 Guide/Example for termination book

Page(s)	Scene/Page description	Purpose
Cover	None	
1	Introduction to therapy (1.2^2)	Introduces protagonist (the child) and setting of the book.
2	Happy time (1.3)	Shares a positive memory.
3	Worry time (2.2)	Indicates reason child came to therapy.
4	Signs of worry (3.1)	Reviews somatic/physiological symptoms of anxiety.
5	Physiological arousal and relaxation	Reviews relaxation techniques.
6–9	Vet visit (5.2)	Reviews Self-talk and anxious thought patterns. Usually requires three to four pictures. Includes information about interventions used through play.
10	Mountain of Worry (6.3)	Usually child draws and relabels mountain on this page. Reviews lessons from session 6.
11	Music group (7.2) or other generic anxiety stem from middle of therapy	Depicts a scene in which child effectively managed anxiety through play.
12–18	Child-specific scenes	Depict additional scene(s) in which child demonstrated effective anxiety management.
19	Wrap-up	Wraps up book by noting ways child has improved during therapy and expresses confidence that similar skills can be used in future.
20	Picture of child and therapist	Final page. Contains farewell statement. Promotes Object permanence of therapist.

also leaves plenty of space to attach 4 × 5 inch photos. In the example below, I have amended the spacing to better fit this book, and I have opted to describe photos, rather than place them, again to conserve space.

This sample termination book describes my work with Gunner,[3] a seven-year-old boy who presented with anxiogenic somatoform symptoms, triggered by school and familial stress. There was also some worry related to security – getting robbed, car being stolen, etc. – despite Gunner living in a fairly safe community, with a low crime rate. He did have one traumatic exposure that precipitated and seemed to explain his security-related worries. His family experienced a total loss of their home during a major storm, which occurred while they were away. However, two pets were inside, both of whom died in the destruction. One pet appeared to have likely been killed instantly by a falling beam. The other pet, though, seemed to have attempted an escape and drowned in the family's pool. Gunner did not show symptoms of PTSD or other traumatic stress disorder, though, from this experience. Rather, his symptoms and presentation were more consistent with general anxious distress, manifesting primarily through stomach aches and headaches (and medical workup suggested these were likely anxiogenic), and, as noted, security-related worries.

As we will see in the example, Gunner's core psychodynamic needs that contributed most to his anxiety were 1) analgesia/need for comfort; 2) loss of love anxiety – in this case, disapproval from parents; and 3) a similar need for approval from other, non-primary caregivers (popularity needs).

Gunner's termination book is described below, along with some general commentary. The text reads exactly as it would in the actual book. Gunner's name is used because the book is about Gunner, so Gunner would be reading about himself in the third person.

Page 1 – space for a photo of activity 1.2 showing a doctor toy sitting in front of Gunner's Self-toy

This is the first day I met Gunner! He was very friendly! When I met Gunner, he was having tummy aches a lot at school. He also had some worry about bad things happening to his family, like getting robbed or their car getting stolen. A lot of people get tummy aches and headaches because they are stressed out. I think that Gunner was having tummy aches because he was a little stressed out at the time about school and about worrying about his home when he was gone to school.

Note, here I am setting the scene and naming the problem.

Page 2 – space for a picture of the Happy time scene

Next, Gunner showed me a happy time. Gunner's happy time was a school scene where Gunner played as the teacher. Gunner played as the teacher and had fun telling all the students what to do. Like a lot of boys, Gunner put a lot of action in his play. In this case, the teacher spanked some of the students and flushed them down the toilet. I think Gunner was showing me in a fun way that he knows that sometimes adults get frustrated and mad at kids.

Here, I am revisiting the Happy time scene, sharing a positive memory. However, I am also recalling a useful insight gathered from my analysis of the scene. In Gunner's story, he depicted an adult character having to intervene somewhat aggressively to rein in unruly children. This scene hinted at something I would see again in Gunner's play, that his personal archetype for "children" is that children play and don't always follow rules, while his archetype for "adult" is one who punishes children when they don't follow rules.

Page 3 – space for a picture here

In this scene, Gunner played the father of a boy who kept trying to "snoop" around the house. Dad was planning a secret trip and he hid the secret in his desk. The boy kept snooping in the desk to find the secret, and the boy got in trouble for sneaking around at night. Like the last scene, in this one, I think Gunner was telling me that sometimes kids do things that are against the rules and they get in trouble for it. Gunner played the Dad in this story, and Gunner showed me in this story that Dads can sometimes punish you, but it doesn't mean they don't love you. Dad forgave his son for snooping, and in the end they went on their secret trip and had a great time!

This scene depicts a major worry of Gunner's, which repeats his conceptualization described on page 2, that adults disapprove when children break rules. However, this time, there is a difference. We are already introducing therapeutic material by helping Gunner finish this story in a therapeutic manner, resolving that even though the Dad did not approve of the child's behaviors, the Dad does still love the child. Further, we see that the reason the Dad was keeping secrets from the child in the first place was in the child's own interest – a surprise trip. So, there is also some acknowledgement here that, yes, sometimes adults keep secrets from children, but there may be a good reason for this. So, the secrecy in this case is not due to a lack of trust or because of a "break" in the relationship. Rather, it is a reflection of care and love for the child.

Page 4 – space for picture of the Robber scene here

This is the Robber scene. In this story, some bad people are trying to steal from a family. We used this story to teach Gunner what happens to the body when people get scared – their hearts beat fast, they can't catch their breath, they sweat, their muscles get tense, and they get sick to their stomach. Gunner said he feels these things when he gets scared too!

On this page, I am reviewing the physiology of anxiety, which is key to Gunner, given his presenting problem.

Page 5 – this page is only text

Now that we know that people's bodies do crazy things when they are scared, nervous, or worried, we had to learn something that would help Gunner's body get back to normal if those things ever happened to his. That's when we started exercising at the beginning of every session. We did the exercise because we wanted to get our hearts beating fast and our blood pumping hard, a lot like what happens to people when they are scared. After we exercised, then we started to tell stories about relaxing. Gunner came up with lots of relaxing stories, and sometimes we used puppets too. In every story, we talked about what Gunner saw, heard, smelled, felt, or even tasted. We went to some place relaxing or happy in our minds and stayed there until we felt relaxed.

We also learned about the "Righty Tighty, Lefty Loosey" game. I taught Gunner this game so that he could practice loosening up his muscles. The more Gunner practices, the better he gets at helping his body relax. I told Gunner that this game was especially useful for untying the knots in his stomach or for catching the butterflies inside whenever they started fluttering around.

Having reviewed the physiology of anxiety, we now review how Gunner learned to relax that anxiety. By putting these details in the termination book, we create a more permanent record of these skills for Gunner to revisit later if needed.

Page 6 – picture of Vet visit stem

This next picture shows another story Gunner and I played. This is the one with the three pets going to visit the vet. In this story, there are three sick pets. One is very worried, one is just a little nervous, and the other is not worried at all. This story let Gunner and I talk about how some people feel different levels of anxiety. It also let us see how we can help control anxiety with our thoughts, by replacing our scared thoughts with happier thoughts. Gunner was really good at helping the pets think good thoughts.

A basic review of the Vet visit stem, with a focus on the CBT skill of replacing negative thoughts with positive alternatives.

Page 7 – another photo of the Vet visit

This is the pet who was very worried. He had a lot of scary thoughts like, "What if something is really wrong with me?" "What if I'm dying?" "What if he gives me a shot?" and so on. Even though his family told him he would be alright, he still couldn't stop himself from having worried thoughts. So, the doctor had to help the dog stop worrying.

Here, we subtly allude to a core need, Gunner's analgesia needs, and his fear of harm.

Page 8 – a third photo of the Vet visit

Gunner came up with an idea to give the dog a bowl of food that would help him feel better. We also decided that maybe if his family were close by, he wouldn't feel so scared. The doctor also put a special medicine in the food that would let the dog stop his worried thoughts and have good thoughts instead. After all of that, the dog began to feel better. The dog didn't have any more worried thoughts. Now, he thought, "That wasn't so bad." "I think I'll be alright." And, "I'm so glad my family is here with me."

This page more explicitly describes the resolution of Gunner's core psycho-dynamic needs. In actual sessions, Gunner offered food to the dog as a way to help calm anxiety. This represented both a gesture of trust – the vet is a friend and will not hurt the dog – and an act of nurturance – "if you have a need, I will fill it." Having family close by helps resolve the loss of love/Object fears that Gunner projected in earlier play, a reminder that he is loved and not alone. Offering medicine is a metaphor for control. By taking the medicine, the dog regained control over worry. It reinforced that Gunner has power/authority over his own mind, and, consequently, over his anxiety.

Page 9

Hey, you know what I just realized! Maybe sometimes when Gunner gets upset, he also has scared thoughts like the dogs did at the vet. Gunner has some nervous thoughts about getting ready to move to Texas. Maybe he thinks, "Will I like my new house?" or, "What if my new teacher isn't like my teacher now?" or, "What if the other kids don't like me?" Hmmmmmm? I wonder what could help Gunner have happier thoughts?

Now, we return to the manifest thoughts characterizing Gunner's anxiety. Again, we return to his fear of harm/discomfort, referencing worries about whether he will like his house (a "discomfort/displeasure" anxiety) and worry about whether others will like him. Now, having worked on love/primary attachment Object needs, we are starting to see some of Gunner's popularity needs.

At the bottom of this page, Gunner was given an option to write in or draw some ideas about what could help him with these thoughts, thereby actively working again in session to reinforce resolution of these needs, even at termination.

Page 10

To figure out what could help, we climbed this Mountain of Worry together. On the mountain, Gunner labeled all the things that upset him. Then, we built steps to climb the mountain that would help Gunner climb over his worries. On the steps, we labeled all the things that help Gunner relax. Are these all the things that help? Or can you think of more?

On this page, I drew a mountain on the page during preparation of the book, with the idea that Gunner and I would repeat an abbreviated form of the activity, labeling a few worries on the mountain, and then also labeling again things that would help. We labeled them together in session.

By adding the text "Are these all the things that help?" we are leaving room for Gunner to review the book later in life, perhaps with family, and he can be prompted to consider additional ideas then, as it is common for preferred coping skills to change over time.

Within an Object-relational framework, we are focusing on the Self on this page, working to reinforce Gunner's confidence in the Self. We are also, again, addressing his dunamis *needs, giving him a sense of power over his own mind.*

Page 11

By now, Gunner is doing better with his feelings. He still gets upset from time to time. Everyone does! But now he really knows how to handle his feelings whenever they do happen. The last few weeks, I noticed his stories aren't about feelings of worry anymore. Now, he plays just like most healthy boys his age play. He makes stories with a lot of action, with good guys against bad guys. Gunner likes to always make sure the good guys win in his stories. This is a good sign, because it means Gunner tells himself that there are happy endings. I bet sometimes he even thinks about his own happy ending. What do you think will be Gunner's happy ending?

This is the only text on this page. On the next page (see below), I left space for Gunner to draw his happy ending.

Page 12

Gunner's happy ending.

Page 13

Gunner is ready to graduate, so here is one last story. In this story, a gorilla family that has lived in the zoo for a while is getting released back into the wild. They have learned everything the zoo can teach them and now they are ready to live on their own back with the other gorillas. The gorillas say goodbye to all of their friends at the zoo, and the zookeepers spend the last night sleeping on top of the gorillas' cage (see them in the picture), so they can be close to them. After saying goodbye, the gorillas go live in the wild where they are happy! They still remember the zookeepers every now and then though. And the zookeepers remember the gorillas too.

This page is designed to revisit our termination session, in preparation to close the book.

Page 14

I think this story is just like Gunner. He has learned everything he needs. I also think that Gunner is very good now at understanding that a little bit of bad feelings is okay and normal for kids, and that he knows exactly what to do if those feelings do get too big – he can use those same steps he has used throughout this book!

And that is how this story about Gunner ends. Gunner may have some things that he will worry about in the future, because EVERYONE worries about something some time or another, but Gunner now knows exactly how to deal with worry, and he has shown me that he is very good at dealing with worry when it does happen!

If Gunner ever forgets, I hope this book can remind him how strong he is.

Page 15

And finally, I have one last picture! This is a picture of Gunner and me from the last time we saw each other! I know I will keep thinking of Gunner every once in a while, even if we don't keep seeing each other. I am proud to have known him!

This page helps promote Object permanence of the therapist, by allowing Gunner to keep a picture of us. By recalling the relationship through this photo, Gunner may be more likely to also recall the lessons of therapy.

Notes

1 Once you have created one book, you will end up with a repository of photos and descriptions from generic story stems that can be used across multiple termination books.
2 Here, activities are coded by session number, then activity number. Session 1, activity 2, then, is coded as 1.2. Session 2, activity 3 would be 2.3, and so on.
3 Name and some details changed to preserve anonymity.

Chapter 11

Creating your own story stems

An essential competence for FELT therapists is building skill in creating therapeutic story stems to fit their clients' needs. In this chapter, I will review guidelines on how to create targeted story stems, for use in particular in the latter half of FELT. Some story stem templates were provided in Chapter 8, and these templates can be used freely as applicable for targeted stems with children who may benefit from them. However, all children have different interests and different needs; so it is essential to be able to create individualized story stems to fit those needs.

What makes a story therapeutic?

There are many kinds of stories. Some were written for entertainment, some for satire, some for political commentary, some for spiritual development, and some for mental development. One important consideration in discussing therapeutic stories, though, is that the impact of a story is a feature not of the author's *intent* but of the *reader's reaction* to the story. So, a story written purely for comedic value can become therapeutic if the reader, having read/heard the comedic story, experiences a beneficial psycho-emotional impact from the story. Thus, in FELT a therapeutic story is defined to be one that *generates or stimulates in the recipient of the story a change that either minimizes the risk of later psychological impairment or boosts overall psychological health (based on the best available, current evidence base), even if only temporarily.*

By this definition, any story, even ones that are just purely entertaining, can be therapeutic, simply by creating a temporary lift in mood. However, the relative "therapeuticness" of a story does vary. A story that provides five minutes of entertainment is unlikely to be as therapeutic as a story that connects deeply with the reader/listener and "sticks" with them in meaningful ways. So, in FELT, therapists must work to prepare stories that maximize the "therapeuticness" of the stories. There are several key components that evidence supports as being likely to boost the therapeutic potential of a story.

DOI: 10.4324/9781032693187-13

One component of therapeuticness is a story's *relational familiarity* (see Mills & Crowley, 1986). Relational familiarity in this context refers to a story's ability to evoke a connection between some component of the story and some aspect of the reader/listener's actual, real-life experiences. Often, relational familiarity occurs through connection with a character, where the reader/listener can see within the character some familiar aspects of themselves or of some other important figure in their life. Relational familiarity, though, can also occur with settings or events within the story. People tend to be drawn to stories that evoke relational familiarity for them. There is a natural affinity for that which is familiar. This is even true for people for whom the familiar aspects have negative connotations. A person who has endured the strife of extreme poverty may not always enjoy stories that remind them of what life is like for people who live in extreme poverty, but most such people do report an interest in such stories, even if for no other reason than to simply "see what it is about," and, presumably, to find out if it connects in any way with their actual experience. It is healthy, in fact, to seek relational familiarity in stories, giving humans a way to process their own experiences through an external lens, and, in many cases, to find inspiration through the characters or events in the story.

I wrote previously in Chapter 3 about proximal and distal influences in Self-development, and how distal influences, even fictional ones, can have a profound impact on a person's sense of Self, especially during childhood. This concept applies here as well. Humans will often seek distal influences to broaden their view of what the world is like. Because distal influences in stories can broaden a person's world view, they can also change, in meaningful ways, a person's psychological makeup, which, in turn, gives those stories the potential to be therapeutic, if the change is beneficial. Some distal influences are not beneficial though. In fact, some can be harmful. Celebrity culture is an example of this. The lure of being rich, beautiful, and famous can easily lead many youth (and adults too) to become enamored with attention, such that they become obsessed with that attention and potentially go to great lengths to "win" it. While it is not inherently unhealthy to enjoy attention from others, the *obsession* with attention can cause people to neglect other aspects of their Self-development and can leave them, as a result, wanting for more than they can ever satisfy. This would all be a result of distal influences touting the incredible and blessed life of celebrity. So, broadening one's world view through distal influences is not always therapeutic, simply by virtue of the fact that a broad view opens up one's mind to both positive and negative influences in the world. If the mind attracts to positive images, then the change is therapeutic. If the mind binds to more negative examples, then the change can become harmful.

Our goal, then, in telling therapeutic stories is to broaden the world view in such a way that positive images overwhelm the negative ones, such that although there is a realization that negative images abound, there is also an acknowledgement that positive examples can balance or even outweigh the negative. **So, a truly therapeutic story does not whitewash the negative aspects of the world. Rather, it recognizes them while giving relatable examples of characters who face negativity and come out of it changed for the better.**

For this reason, all stories that FELT therapists create contain a moment of "tension," a point in which the rest of the story can go either way – good or bad – depending on the choices of the characters (and of the narrator). This tension point is almost always where story *stems* end and where children take over in helping to finish the stories. In creating stories, therapists have infinite possibilities about where to create the tension point. However, there are some additional guidelines for setting up a tension point to maximize its efficacy with any particular client.

Choosing a tension point

There are four key factors to consider in choosing a tension point for story stems you create for your child client. We consider each of these individually below.

1) What are the child's skills for managing tension at this stage in treatment?
Ideally, a child's readiness to manage tension increases over the course of treatment. The generic story stems are written and progress as they do under the assumption that, at the beginning of treatment, abilities to resolve high tension are relatively weak. This is why the first session contains no real tension in story stems and why the second session contains a very low stress stem. By session 3, tension levels begin to increase, but do so in ways that are unlikely to be realistic for most (i.e., the Robber stem depicts a low-likelihood event for most children; the Vet visit in session 5 uses animals, instead of people, to create additional relational distance). Still, as FELT progresses, generic story stems increase in their likelihood both for relational familiarity and for creating a realistic tension for children. Once the child progresses to a stage of using targeted story stems – those which you create as a therapist – they are likely to have already built some basic skills for managing that tension. Still, you should always ask yourself before creating a stem whether the child is where they should (are expected to) be with regard to tension reduction in story stems so far. If a child has needed a lot of support in previous stems, you may choose to create a relatively "weak" stem, more amenable to their current skill set. If a child seems particularly strong, you may choose to challenge them a bit more directly a bit earlier than you would other children.

2) What level of relational familiarity can they handle?
Following similarly from the first principle above, you should also consider a child's relative readiness for varying levels of relational familiarity. Tension and relational familiarity, in fact, are inseparably bound to each other, such that, for a clinically anxious child, relational familiarity increases tension and

increased tension causes increased relational familiarity. So, as story stems progressively increase in tension, the tension itself sparks a familiarity with the tension children feel when they become anxious. If the tension itself is the only level of familiarity, children early in therapy are typically more tolerant of this than if you are to begin the first session with an exact replication of the child's most anxiety-provoking moment. So, one way FELT therapists manage tension is by managing familiarity of the story stems. To maximize therapeuticness, early story stems should have *some* relational familiarity, but typically familiarity is minimized to one to three components. As therapy progresses, and as you get to know the child better as therapist, you can introduce increasing levels of familiarity until eventually you and the child are essentially playing out real-world scenarios during session. So, just like with tension, when creating your own story stems, you should consider how much familiarity to introduce based on how far along you are in therapy and how well the child has managed previous increasing levels of familiarity.

3) What are important themes learned from early sessions that can be included and/or manipulated as needed in creating targeted story stems?

As a FELT therapist, your case formulation – using the FELT etiological model – forms the key basis upon which you create targeted story stems. In fact, it is impossible to create a truly therapeutic story stem without first having a good, detailed case formulation. Early sessions are designed specifically in part to give you a baseline about what is familiar to the child and about what toys, characters, and scenes they identify with. By the time a child reaches the second phase of FELT, they will have undergone numerous story stems and numerous scenarios, which are "grist for the mill" of creating individualized story stems in the latter half of FELT. So, when creating individualized story stems, it is important to take an inventory of your previous sessions with the child and consider what kinds of characters and events that child connects to. Does your client tend to connect better with animal characters versus human characters? How do they depict "home" in play – is home a place of shelter? If so, how can "home" be used in individualized stories as a potential safe base when facing targeted anxieties? When addressing anxiety, do children tend to prefer certain coping mechanisms over others? If your client in early sessions has turned often toward others for help, how can you write stories such that others are still available to provide help if needed? Or, on the contrary, to help boost or teach a better diversity of coping skills, should you create stories that limit a "favorite" coping skill? If the child has previously relied heavily on others to offer comfort when distressed, should you consider creating stories where they must manage stress with less intervention from others, as a means to boost familiarity with a wider range of coping skills? In whatever way you choose to use it, information from early sessions forms a vital repository of data from which to create targeted stems.

4) What is the "core" problem you want to address with this story? Think deeper than the manifest factors of the anxiety. Think instead about the propagating factors. How can you create a story that gives the child an opportunity to resolve propagating factors?

Among the most important tenets of FELT is the focus on creating therapeutic interventions toward propagating factors, rather than just manifest anxiety. Generalized story stems necessarily focus primarily on manifest factors, using play-based exposures and practice to modulate overt symptoms of negative affect and autonomic arousal. The primary goal of targeted story stems, however, is to address individualized propagating factors associated with each child's anxiety. Because they focus on the individual domain (rather than the environmental or biological domain), psychodynamic factors become paramount in generating maximally therapeutic story stems (as outlined previously, environmental factors are typically addressed outside of individual therapy). So, when planning and creating targeted FELT story stems, it is of absolute importance to first create a strong dynamic formulation of the core problem contributing to the manifest anxiety. What human need is not being met/resolved healthily in this child? Based on your dynamic formulation, you will then create/select targeted story stems to address the unmet dynamic need.

In the sections below, I review two detailed examples of the creation of a targeted stem to address a specific problem in therapy.

Example 1: Jane creates a story to address dunamis fear

Jane (therapist) has worked with Bryan (age six) for eight weeks/sessions in FELT. Bryan presented initially to therapy with symptoms consistent with uncomplicated Separation Anxiety Disorder. Over the course of therapy so far, Bryan has progressed well through treatment. In fact, he even reports minimal separation anxiety now, and he is able to tolerate separations from both parents without significant distress. From a symptom perspective, Bryan appears to be ready to terminate sessions; however, a dynamic analysis of Bryan's previous eight therapy sessions suggests a recurring theme that his separation anxiety appears predicted by a consistent *dunamis* fear. In other words, Bryan's play consistently shows him to be a passive character in resolving tension states. Things get resolved in play, yes, but almost never does the resolution have anything to do with something Bryan has done. Instead, he is always rescued by an outside force, dependent on others to save him. The ongoing presence of this fear puts Bryan at risk for challenges should his separation anxiety (or any other anxiety, for that matter) re-emerge. So, Jane, as therapist, elects to work with Bryan to build a stronger sense of confidence in his own potential and ability to resolve tension states, thus helping to resolve his unmet *dunamis* need.

To facilitate developing a stronger sense of *dunamis*, Jane decides to create a story stem where the main character must rescue themselves. She first takes inventory of Bryan's previous sessions and remembers that he often seems to identify with weaker, helpless characters in play, often depicting his Self-toy as a small animal being attacked by predators. Jane decides to recreate a similar scene, using animals Bryan is familiar with. She first chooses characters: a bunny, a lion, and an alligator. With characters selected, Jane can now start to consider story lines. The first story that comes to mind involves a pet bunny who gets separated from its owners in the wild. This feels like a good start because it also highlights some of Bryan's separation anxiety. Given Bryan's separation anxiety at home seems now well managed, Jane feels that Bryan can handle a more intense story stem about separation anxiety, so she purposely chooses not to introduce the bunny's owners into the story stem, and she decides that even if Bryan wants to bring them in, she will not allow it until the bunny has worked to provide its own sense of security (that is, Jane may allow the bunny to return home at the end of the story, but only after the bunny has dealt with the sense of insecurity present when it was lost in the wild).

Next, Jane must consider where to leave a tension point for the bunny. Jane's stem idea for the bunny is very similar to the lost baby elephant story stem played in session 7, so she already has some information from that stem about how Bryan may be likely to respond in this stem. In the lost baby elephant stem, Bryan had the mother elephant come find the baby, a passive response for the baby, who did nothing to help mother find it or to provide security while lost. So, in this story, Jane wants the bunny to take a more active role in handling tension. She first considers having the lion and the alligator surround the bunny with seemingly no way out, but Jane feels this may be too big a challenge for Bryan, and not realistic. It would not be healthy for a six-year-old to be left alone and feel they had to fend for themselves against terroristic threats from dangerous predators. So, Jane considers a story that is more realistic for his age and not overly intense for young Bryan. After thoughtful consideration, Jane decides that it is perfectly reasonable to expect six-year-old children to solve some challenges on their own (with proper scaffolding, of course) and that they commonly do so at school, with tests. She decides to mimic this with a story about "passing trials" to return home, a story line likely to be familiar to children, as it is commonly used in children's stories.

Thus, in the story Jane created, she sets up a scene where the bunny is lost in the wilderness and must find its own way back home. But, to get home, it must face two trials: the trial of the swamp and the trial of the Sahara. First comes the trial of the swamp. In the story, Jane tells of the trial of the swamp, which is offered by the alligator. The alligator stands at the swamp and tells the bunny about the challenge: "Hello! Welcome to the trial of the swamp! Your task is to get to the other side with only four hops. If you take more than four hops, I will grab you in my mouth and take you back to the start, where you can try again. If you want to get back home to your family though, you must pass this trial." Jane then demonstrates how to solve the trial by analyzing the problem, taking deep breaths to stay relaxed, and then jumping across lily pads. For some narrative flair, she adds a fancy trapeze-like move to allow the bunny to technically cover a lot of ground in fewer hops. The bunny gets to the other side and celebrates before moving on to the next trial, the trial of the Sahara. In this challenge, the bunny must endure one full night alone in the Sahara, and then the lion will let the bunny pass. The lion promises to protect the bunny from afar and that even though the bunny will not see the lion, the lion will not let it be killed by any other wild animals. The lion does warn that if the bunny runs away from the specified spot, it must go back and try again another night. At this point, Jane turns the story over to Bryan, asking: "What happens next?"

The story example highlights well the key features of creating a targeted story stem to address a specific problem. It is a direct analogue of separation anxiety, which attacks the symptom domain. It is also, though, structured specifically to help Bryan build a stronger sense of independence and power, a key weakness according to Bryan's formulation, by learning to solve "trials" on his own. Likewise, the story takes into consideration Brian's developmental stage and seeks to create some realism in expectations. Even though the story content itself is fantastical and non-realistic (a six-year-old would hopefully never be left alone in the Sahara), it mimics the real problem on two levels: 1) there is actual separation from "parents" (owners), and 2) the bunny must spend a night alone without being able to see the guardian (lion). As such, the bunny must learn to trust the Object permanence of the absent guardians to provide safety, and the bunny must learn to reassure itself that it is safe, even if it does feel frightened – that the feeling of insecurity does not reflect reality. Thus, the metaphor reflects a common reality of childhood and gives Bryan a chance to resolve those issues in a healthy manner. Lastly, in creating the story, Jane considered Bryan's readiness for such a stem and used scaffolding in the story stem to give him some guidance in what needed to be accomplished. If she felt Bryan were ready for it, Jane could have had him complete both trials on his own during the session, rather than only the second, and then could have collaborated or set limits as needed to ensure he met the goal of building *dunamis* power through play.

Example 2: Chris addresses superego needs

Chris (therapist) has worked with Dara (age eight) for seven weeks in FELT. Dara's original presenting complaint was a generalized anxiety, characterized by over-worrying with panic attacks. Dara's panic attacks were triggered frequently at school, when she had to take "big tests." During state-required benchmark testing last year, Dara broke down in tears, began to feel sick to her stomach, and hyperventilated, causing her to have to see the school nurse. This prompted Dara's referral to psychotherapy, and a clinical interview revealed significant performance anxiety at school, but also more generalized worries, including almost obsessive worry about parents (specifically, Dara worried about her parents' finances, who, though not living in poverty, per se, did complain at times about needing to be careful with how they spend money). Though she was a well-behaved child, she also often worried about "getting in trouble" or "doing things wrong."

In FELT, Chris had already worked with Dara and achieved good progress in several areas. Symptoms of panic were diminished, but worry continued. In particular, Chris noted through session content that Dara seemed to have considerable superego anxiety. In other words, much of the pressure she felt about "doing things wrong" or "getting a bad grade" came internally. Her parents did not put any pressure on her for good grades, and genuinely did not care about grades; they genuinely only cared that Dara enjoyed school and seemed to be learning (which she was – academically, her grades were consistently good, As and Bs). Dara seemed to have developed this internal sense that she had to be perfect, which Chris recognized as a manifestation of superego anxiety.[1] For the next session, he wanted to create a targeted story stem to allow Dara to work through this superego anxiety in more detail.

Chris knew from previous sessions that Dara had latched heavily onto princess toys. When given the choice, Dara almost always incorporated princesses from a well-known cartoon-maker. Chris decided to create a story using these princesses. He set up the following scene for Dara.

"Ella invited all her princess friends to her birthday party. She was so excited to have all her friends come over to her house, but she was also a little stressed out, and she worried everything would go wrong. She planned many fun activities. Over here, she has pony rides. In the kitchen, she has a 'make your own cupcake' bar. There is also a bouncy house and a courtyard where you can talk to forest animals. Finally, in Ella's bedroom, she set up a dance and karaoke party. Still, the day of the party, Ella started to panic a little. She feels like she still hasn't done enough and can't shake the feeling that something will go wrong. Her parents keep telling her that 'Everything will be alright,' but she doesn't believe it. She's getting more and more nervous, and then, suddenly, the doorbell rings and three of her friends arrive at the same time. What happens next?"

Chris also specifically plans ahead to push Dara's limits a bit in the session, dragging the scene out as needed to allow Dara multiple challenges to address through the session. He wants to offer Dara an early opportunity to collaborate in the stem, so he keeps the initial stem short, but he also plans additional "parts" of the story which he can use as needed depending on how Dara responds. In fact, Chris imagines something that can go slightly wrong with each of the "stations" at the party. With the ponies, Chris plans to make one of them be rather uncooperative, refusing to be ridden and refusing to go in the right direction. At the cupcake station, Chris plans to have one princess ask if there is any "caramel syrup" to use, but Ella does not have any. At the bouncy house, only three girls will be allowed at one time, no exceptions, and for the courtyard, three of the princesses won't be interested because they have their own pets at home and don't feel like talking to animals today. Lastly, at the dance and karaoke party, Ella will not have one of the songs that one of the princesses wanted to sing "very badly." By layering the story in this way, Chris creates multiple opportunities and challenges for Ella to face in session, and through all of them, Chris specifically wants to highlight Ella's own superego anxiety. Consequently, he also plans to use prompts if needed to ensure that Dara addresses superego thoughts. If needed, Chris plans to narrate Ella's thoughts and highlight her superego anxiety. For example, as more and more "problems" arise during the party, Ella says to herself, "Ugghh, nothing is going right. It's all my fault. Why can't I do anything right?" Chris hopes this narration will prompt Dara to produce a therapeutic response of her own through the play, but if it does not, he is prepared to prompt further by reminding Dara how to "fight" worried thoughts.

Multilayered stories

The story examples above provide useful depictions of another advanced FELT technique: multilayered therapeutic stories. Whereas early and generic story stems are often designed to address specific, singular issues/skills, later, targeted stories can often become multilayered and sectioned to address multiple skills and/or to allow repetitive exposure to a therapeutic topic. In Example 1, Jane used a multilayered story to prime Bryan toward the desired therapeutic response, but she could have just as easily allowed Bryan to play through both sections of the story, to promote better mastery. In Example 2, Chris prepared numerous challenges to help Dara master the skill of challenging her perfectionist ideas. Multilayered stories are an efficient way to allow repetition of a therapeutic concept without having to stop/tear down a scene and start/build a new one. Thus, FELT therapists are encouraged to create multilayered stories when possible to allow sessions to progress more seamlessly.

Multilayered stories can also be used to address different therapeutic needs. Example 3 below provides a sample of a multilayered story to address both *exousia* needs and the need for love.

Example 3: Brett creates a story to simultaneously address needs for exousia *and for love*

Brett (therapist) is working with Jeanie (age nine) on performance anxiety. Jeanie becomes so terrified of speaking in front of her class that she started to purposely perform below her ability so that she would not have to participate in the class speech project. She not only purposely wrote a poor speech, but she also began "tanking" her other writing assignments so that the teacher would be less likely to "nominate" her to participate in the school-wide speech contest. Importantly, Jeanie is generally a high achiever in all-academic areas, and school is easy for her. So, the fact that she is purposely performing below her ability in writing is out of character for her. When her parents noticed her low grades and asked her about them, she revealed to them her anxiety about the contest, and they brought her to see Brett for counseling.

Having worked with Jeanie for some time, Brett developed a formulation that her performance anxiety was built heavily around *exousia* and loss of love needs. Jeanie believed that if she performed badly on the speech in front of her class, she would lose some of her "standing" with her peers as the "smart girl." She was proud of being smart and being smart was an important part of her identity. It gave her a sense of authority in her world, that if she was the "smart" girl, she could be anything. It also made her feel others trusted her opinion, and she convinced herself that if she gave a bad speech to the whole school, none of her friends would ask her for help on school anymore. Additionally, Jeanie also feared that if she wasn't "smart," her parents would not be proud of her anymore either. She reasoned that if she got bad grades on purpose, it would not be due to a lack of ability, whereas if she failed while trying her best, this would mean she was not actually "smart." So, she felt okay failing on purpose. This way, her failure was not a true failure; rather, it was a conscious defense against having to give a public speech.

Brett recognized these features as being representative of *exousia* fears and loss of love fears. So, in working with Jeanie, he needed to develop stories that addressed these fears. Having progressed to an advanced stage of psychotherapy, Brett wanted to prepare a multilayered story to target each of these fears within the same story. Brett began his creative process by first considering a scene that may trigger *exousia* and loss of love needs. Brett knew from his education on developmental psychology that both of these human needs are activated during toddlerhood, especially during separation-individuation stages of toddlerhood, where toddlers test the limits of their own authority and independence, while still needing parents to stay present and care for them. Thus, Brett decided to create a story that mimicked the separation-individuation stage of toddlerhood. He knew that Jeanie liked playing with animal characters, so he also decided to use animal characters in the scene. Out of convenience, he chose to use a gorilla family, because his toy collection included two gorilla parents and one young gorilla. Lastly, since Jeanie's real-world problem involved fear of underperforming to her ability, Brett wanted in particular to capture the complex *exousia* fears present in Jeanie's Self-identity not matching with her feared performance on the speech. He felt it would not connect as well simply to enact toddler-like defiance as an exercise of *exousia* authority. Instead, he needed to create a detailed enough character backstory to give the toddler gorilla in this case a similar type of identity-based fear to that experienced by Jeanie.

Given the above considerations, Brett elected to make the toddler gorilla be an excellent climber. In fact, the toddler gorilla was "the best young climber in the whole troop" of gorillas. Further, Brett outlined that the toddler gorilla's parents were particularly proud of her climbing ability (Brett purposely made toddler gorilla a female in this case, to better match Jeanie's own gender identity). The parents would often bring their daughter to some of the tallest trees in the jungle to practice climbing and they would give her challenges that other young gorillas did not get. Every time, though, the young gorilla would rise to the challenge and climb all the tallest trees. All her friends would always pat her on the back and congratulate her when they saw how good a climber she was. Brett would also specify in the backstory that the young gorilla even became the *authority* (a word he would be sure to use often during the story stem with Jeanie, given her formulation) on climbing among all the young gorillas in the troop. Other gorillas would often ask her for help on their climbing, and she would often teach others her techniques for climbing. In fact, this was something she was most *proud* of, being *trusted* by others to *coach* them in her skill.

With this backstory established, Brett can move toward the story stem. In the stem, Brett sets up a troop of gorillas, but he also sets up all the other jungle animals he can find, telling Jeanie that they were invited to see the troop perform their climbs. Brett also makes a point to place the protagonist gorilla's parents in the front row, and they even brought a camera to record it. They bragged to their friends and even told some of the other jungle animals they'd never met before that their daughter was an excellent climber and that they were "so excited" to see her performance. Brett notes that the troop of young gorillas were nervous at the idea of having to perform in front of the rest of the jungle. Even the expert climber was nervous. In fact, she seemed most nervous of everyone, because she felt the *most pressure* to do well, because everyone expected her to do so well. Brett ends the story stem with the following statement: "The young gorilla got so nervous that she even worried if she should go through with the climb. She thought, 'What if I just don't show up? Or if I pretend to be sick so I don't have to climb?' What happens next?"

With this story stem, Brett first identified *exousia* and loss of love needs. In creating the story, he set the story to occur during toddlerhood, a time when those particular needs are normatively quite active in children. However, as the story developed in Brett's mind, the fact that the young gorilla was a toddler mattered little to the actual story, and the story could have proceeded identically with an older gorilla. Setting in toddlerhood, then, became more of a choice based on psychodynamic and developmental theory that *exousia* and loss of love needs are important to resolve during toddlerhood, and he wanted to give Jeanie a chance to reflect (albeit perhaps subconsciously) on the possibility that her own current fears may have a longer history than just now at this debate. Of course, he would not expect Jeanie to reflect openly on this history in psychotherapy, as doing so would be inconsistent with normal age expectations. Even though such a technique may be used in adult psychoanalysis, it would not be appropriate for Brett to invite Jeanie to self-analyze the origins of her fears. Instead, he wants to activate them through play and allow her a chance to resolve them in healthy ways, again, through that same play. By giving Jeanie an opportunity to resolve this gorilla stem, he opens her up to generalization of the skill outside of therapy and helps her reach a place where she is more likely to resolve the core of the presenting problem, her *exousia* and loss of love fears. Furthermore, by repeating this stem (or similar ones) multiple times over the course of FELT, Brett helps Jeanie build stronger mastery over these fears.

A template for story creation

As can be seen from the examples above, and based on my experience in developing FELT and in training others in FELT, a rudimentary template emerged in guiding the creation of new story stems. I outline the template below that has worked well for me and for some of the students and therapists I have trained. However, this template is only one option and is provided for the convenience of those who wish to use it. Different storytellers have different ways of creating the stories they tell, and new FELT therapists are encouraged to find their own methods for building stories, given they still follow the other guidelines outlined with regard to ensuring the stories remain therapeutic.

Step 1: identify a problem to be addressed with the story.

Step 2: survey resources (what toys/supplies are available) to choose what may be used in the story.

Step 3: choose characters. Characters are usually the most important part of FELT stories, because the characters are designed to capture the proper level of relational familiarity with the child. Given their importance, I have found it useful often to start by selecting characters and planning a story around them.

Step 4: with characters chosen, now place the characters in a therapeutically meaningful context. The specific context depends on many factors and the process for developing the context varies across stories and across cases. In some stories, therapists start with the environment they will set up in the scene and will create a story from there. In others, therapists may start with a backstory for the characters (as seen in Example 3), and then create the context of the stem to support the backstory. Sometimes, characters will not even need much of a backstory, with the context of the stem itself capturing everything necessary for therapeutic goals. Whatever the case, step 4 involves taking chosen characters and then creating a basic context either through a surrounding scene or through a backstory.

Step 5: choose a tension point for the story stem, using the guidelines outlined in this chapter.

Step 6: plan additional "layers" to the story as needed. These layers can be implemented during the stem itself or saved as secondary "stems" to introduce during collaborative play. For both, therapists should typically plan where they want stories to go even after the child takes over direction of the play and prepare suggestions to move that play in therapeutic directions as needed. In executing plans, therapists should of course remain flexible and responsive to the child's cues, as outlined elsewhere in this manual.

With these guidelines in mind and with the experience of early FELT sessions behind them, FELT therapists often find themselves becoming quick experts in FELT story creation. As therapists create more stories, a process typically emerges that increases their efficiency. Eventually, expert FELT therapists get so comfortable at story creation that they may even be able to do so "on the spot" in sessions with children, if such an opportunity arises. Still, even in those cases, therapists are always advised to plan stories in advance, as doing so helps ensure a more thoughtful process and allows for more complex storytelling. "On the spot" creation is permitted, but only in certain (rather rare) circumstances, such as with a child who is themselves a rather rich storyteller and who enjoys creating their own stories in session. In such cases, more often than not, children get carried away with introducing more "entertaining" aspects of their stories and tend to be unconcerned with therapeutic storytelling. So, therapists must work in those circumstances to quickly introduce story components to drive the story toward therapeutic avenues. Only experienced FELT therapists, those who have successfully completed four or more cases of executing FELT from start to finish, are typically able to "save" an entertaining (but not therapeutic) child-created story to make it more therapeutic. Less experienced therapists are encouraged instead, if they allow child-created stories at all, to allow them usually only at the ends of sessions, after session goals have been executed, to give children a chance to "just play" and only for a few minutes (no more than ten). Of course, therapists should still follow other FELT guidelines to make child-directed stories as therapeutic as possible, but no FELT session should begin with a general goal of "just letting the child play" and following their lead throughout. Although a completely non-directive approach is one approach to Play Therapy (see Virginia Axline's (1974) work for a prototypical sample), if a therapist finds themselves executing a session without any story stems, they are no longer doing FELT.

Note

1   Perfectionism, in fact, is a common sign of superego anxiety, so much so that its presence should always cue clinicians to consider superego needs.

REFERENCES

Axline, V. M. (1974). *Play Therapy*. New York: Ballantine Books.

Mills, J. C., & Crowley, R. J. (1986). *Therapeutic Metaphors for Children and the Child within*. New York: Brunner/Mazel.

Chapter 12

Future directions

After 12 years in development and dissemination, FELT has shown great promise of efficacy in studies for treating anxiety, and this book has used the example of clinical anxiety to demonstrate how FELT is structured and administered to address anxious symptoms. However, as I have tried to make clear throughout this book, the concepts of FELT can be applied to treat other clinical conditions as well, namely depressive and stressor-related disorders, both of which have known etiological, symptom, and treatment overlap with anxiety disorders. FELT is not supposed to be a treatment for anxiety, but a framework through which therapists can execute evidence-based principles through creative, semi-directive Play Therapy. Consequently, major future directions for FELT including adapting the framework to address the specific etiological models for other clinical syndromes in addition to anxiety. In this chapter, I propose a method through which FELT may be adapted to address depressive disorders, as an example of how FELT may be adapted in the future.

Adapting for depressive disorders

Before reviewing possible applications of FELT in childhood depression, it is first important to define clinical depression. Depressive disorders revolve heavily around definitions of Major Depressive Episodes (MDEs). The presence and persistence of one or more MDEs in a patient's clinical history identifies that patient as having a depressive disorder, either Major Depressive Disorder (single episode or recurrent) or Persistent Depressive Disorder (defined in children as the persistence of major depressive symptoms for at least one year, with no more than a two-month period of symptom relief). The *DSM-5* (American Psychiatric Association, 2013) defines an MDE as the presence of five or more of the following nine symptoms,[1] over at least a two-week period. Importantly, one of the five symptoms must be either 1) depressed mood or 2) anhedonia, below:

1 Depressed mood most of the day, nearly every day,
2 Anhedonia, or decreased pleasure in all or nearly all activities, most of the day, nearly every day,

DOI: 10.4324/9781032693187-14

3   Changes in weight or appetite (increased or decreased, or, in young children, failure to gain weight within normal expectations),
4   Changes in sleep (sleeping more or sleeping less),
5   Restlessness or psychomotor retardation,
6   Fatigue or low energy,
7   Feelings of worthlessness and/or guilt,
8   Trouble concentrating or indecisiveness,
9   Recurrent thoughts of death and/or suicide.

As with all *DSM* disorders, these symptoms should not be better explained by other factors and should cause clinically significant functional impairment.

One problem with this definition of MDEs is that they are based on *adult* and *adolescent* presentations of depressive illness. Children (under ten years old) with depressed mood tend to present differently, and, as a result, rarely meet criteria for MDE as defined in DSM-5. An alternative diagnostic clinical manual for early childhood (ages 0–5), called *Diagnostic Classification of Mental Health and Developmental Disorders of Infancy and Early Childhood*, better known as the *DC:0–5* (Zero to Three, 2016), provides more specificity for early childhood depression. The nine criteria in the *DC:0–5* are the same as those listed in the *DSM-5*, but the text further specifies how these symptoms appear in early childhood. Characteristically, young children do not directly express chronically sad or depressed mood. Rather, these signs are observed by others. Most often, young children who are depressed present with chronic irritability and higher-than-normal frequency of tantrums. Tantrums include aggressive behaviors (e.g., biting, kicking, hitting) and may often be directed at the Self as well (Self-harm).

Anhedonic depression in young children is similar to melancholic depression in adults, characterized by decreased initiation of play with others, psychomotor retardation, and decreased energy. Again, young children rarely express verbally anhedonia; rather, anhedonia is inferred from a change in interest in previously enjoyed activities. At the same time, healthy children quite commonly change interests in activities and may lose interest in things they used to enjoy. Changing interests is therefore developmentally normative and usually not a sign of anhedonia. The ubiquity of normative changes in interests among children is another feature that complicates diagnosis of anhedonia, and, subsequently, depression in young children.

One important feature of early childhood, as noted in Chapter 3, is their tendency toward normal narcissism. Young children like to show off their skills in a proud, almost boastful manner. Although such behavior may be discouraged in adulthood in favor of humility, it is often encouraged in children and is an important part of healthy Self-development. So, the persistent absence of normal narcissism can be a key indicator of depression, especially if that narcissism is instead replaced by Self-deprecation and expressions of worthlessness. Often these symptoms may not be apparent in verbalizations, but may emerge through play.

Even though depression in preschool and elementary-aged children can be identified, it is far less prevalent in young children than in adolescence and young adulthood. The *DC:0–5* gives prevalence estimates of 0.5%–2% in children aged 3–5 years. The rate is far higher in adolescence. According to data from 2019, 15.5% of all US adolescents were diagnosed with at least one MDE that year (Daly, 2022). There is also a well-known "female skew" for depression, with about a 3:1 ratio. So, according to those same 2019 data, 23.4% of females ages 12–17 were diagnosed with an MDE in 2019, compared to 8.4% of adolescent males. Among US adults ages 26–49, the overall rate was 9.3%, and among those over 50, the rate was 4.5%.[2] So, as the data show, young children have the lowest risk among all ages of being diagnosed with depression.

One of the reasons for these low prevalence rates in children is that because children do not verbally express sadness and anhedonia, and because depressed mood presents more often as irritability and with temper tantrums, young children with internal psychological distress are much more likely to be diagnosed with (and treated for) anxiety or stressor-related disorders than depressive disorders. However, there are good clinical data to suggest, perhaps, that diagnostic specificity for depression versus anxiety in children (especially younger children) does not matter (Fitzpatrick et al., 2023). There is great treatment overlap among treatments for depression and anxiety, especially with regard to cognitive behavioral models, and etiological models for both are also quite similar. So, there is an argument that, from a practical perspective, it is enough to simply identify children who need treatment for the presence of negative affect, and then to treat them for it, without worrying too greatly if semantically we call the symptoms depression or anxiety.[3]

Of course, it is important to consider ongoing research differentiating pediatric anxiety from depression, so that new treatments may emerge or so that prognostic data can be more accurate. However, decades of clinical research have supported considerable overlap among diagnoses and treatments of negative affect in children, and so it is perfectly reasonable for practicing clinicians to focus more on treating the specific problems resulting in presentation for clinical services, rather than to focus on treating a diagnosis. Treatments both for depression and for anxiety share several key components. First, although thought content differs between anxiety and depression, treatment approaches for both are linked by their mutual attention to addressing negative thoughts. Similarly, the negative affect present in both anxiety and depression often controls behaviors, such that patients suffering from both disorders feel at the mercy of their mood and affect, unable to move forward. Thus, another shared treatment goal is to help patients identify healthy coping plans to take back control such that they can pursue goals regardless of their emotions. Treatments teach patients not to deny their emotions, but to acknowledge them and regain control over them so that they can pursue other interests.

Despite similarities, there are still differences between anxiety and depression, and though treatments share common key goals, they often work to reach those goals in unique ways, based on specific etiological needs. FELT's etiological framework highlights this individualized approach to treatment planning, where interventions are planned to address specific problems in manifest, propagating, and temporal factors involved in a clinical problem. Though that same structure can be used to treat depression, the propagating, manifest, and temporal factors included in a model of depression would not be the same as those used in anxiety.

The first step, then, to adapt FELT to depression (or any disorder, for that matter) is to first outline a strong etiological model consistent with that outlined in Chapters 6 and 7. Fortunately, decades of clinical research on the etiology of depressive disorders already exists to inform such a model. Perhaps the most widely cited model differentiating depression from anxiety is the PANAAS model, an acronym that stands for Positive Affect, Negative Affect, (and) Autonomic Sensitivity. The PANAAS model posits that anxiety and depression both share high levels of negative affect. Positive affect, however, is typically within normal limits in pure anxiety, whereas it is low in depression. In other words, depressed patients show lower-than-normal rates of positive emotions, whereas those with anxiety still experience plentiful positive emotion; they just also experience plentiful (too much) negative emotion. Autonomic sensitivity tends to be higher in anxiety than in depression, but patients with depression can also have high levels of autonomic sensitivity, especially if there is co-morbid anxiety (which is common). Some patients with depression may show signs of *underarousal*, which can be postulated as a sign of low autonomic sensitivity or autonomic insensitivity. In this form of depression (a more melancholic depression), the patient experiences numbing of emotional sensations, low drive, apathy, and low motivation. They feel almost as if they "can't get going." Those with high autonomic sensitivity, on the other hand, are often "on edge," feel restless, and have plenty of drive, but are too overcome by negative emotionality to pursue drives. So, we can see from the PANAAS model two distinctive features of depression that are not usually present in pure anxiety (that is, anxiety without depression): low positive affect and autonomic underreactivity. As explained earlier, this is one reason depression is rarely diagnosed in young children, because they rarely show the low affect and autonomic underreactivity that define depression. Still, when these problems do present in children, they should be addressed specifically in psychotherapy.

Consequently, any version of FELT adapted for depression would need to include, in its manifest factors, signs of low positive affect and of autonomic underreactivty (e.g., numbing, low drive, flat affect, etc.). Propagating factors would also need amendment. Environmental risk factors for depression are congruent to those found in anxiety and are extensive, so I will not review them again here. Biological factors are also similar, with a focus on various experiences or stimuli that amplify or suppress biological vulnerabilities. The aims of medications (antidepressants) are also similar to those outlined for anxiety in Chapter 7. However, biological aims in treating depression do differ in that there is not usually a goal to promote sedation/de-arousal. Rather, the aim is often the opposite, to promote activation and energy. Propagating factors would differ most greatly in dynamic factors.

A full review of dynamic factors involved in depression is beyond the scope of this book, but I will review a few here as a means to demonstrate some ways FELT for depression may differ from FELT for anxiety. The most classic Freudian explanation of depression, introduced in "Mourning and Melancholia" (Freud, 1917), described depressed affect resulting from real, actual loss (mourning) versus that experienced from *emotional* loss (melancholia). Freud described melancholia as a profound loss of self-esteem, a consequence of Self-deprecation triggered by anger turned inward. So, to Freud, melancholic sadness was a symptom of Self-anger. More specifically, the Self-anger derived from the patient's psychological combination of the Self with a lost Object. The only way they could cope with the loss of an important Object was to blame the Self, which led to depression. Klein (1940) further elaborated that this process of Self-blame contributes to a process of Self-destruction and that Self-destruction, in turn, leads a person to imagine that Others are persecuting them as well. It is for this reason that depressed persons often reason that Others dislike them too. Such pessimistic attitudes about Others derive from Self-destructive anger at the Self.

Not all dynamic theorists believe that depression is a secondary affective state to the primary emotion of anger turned inward. Bibring (1953) was one of the first theorists to write about the primary affective state of depression, and he viewed depression as a result of a mismatch between a person's ideals and their reality. In terms of childhood development, primary depression results from the realization of the limits of a person's normal narcissism and being unable to reconcile those limits with the sense of Self. The awareness that one is not actually as worthy, superior, and perfectly good as their normal narcissism would have them believe leads to a psychological tension that must be relieved by adaptation of the Self. A healthy adaptation would be to recognize that one cannot meet every dream or goal, and that is okay. A depressive adaptation, on the other hand, occurs when a person turns toward guilt and shame about their inability to meet those presupposed ideals. Over time, this adaptation can turn into an internalization of the Self as the "bad object."

Overall, in all psychodynamic theories, depression is a feature of the destruction of the Self in the context of perceived failures in interpersonal relationships. Classically, two types of depression emerge from this Self-destruction. *Anaclitic* depression presents as helplessness, loneliness, and powerlessness at the prospect of being abandoned by Others. Those with anaclitic depression focus on the inevitability of abandonment and loneliness. They long for nurturance from Others, but feel they will never get the love they need.

Introjective depression, on the other hand, is characterized more by unworthiness, failure, inferiority, and guilt. In this case, Self-destructive processes lead the patient to believe that their sense of loneliness and fear of abandonment results from an inherent problem with the Self. In anaclitic depression, the problem is with the inevitability of loneliness. In introjective depression, the problem is that person feels they, themselves, are not worthy of love, and even though love is available to others, it will never be available to them.

To use the dynamic model outlined in FELT, then, treatment of depression would focus on the human needs for love and for Objects and would seek to explore possible unresolved tension with those needs in the treatment of depressed children. So, a child may express they feel sad because they "do not have any friends." This statement would prompt the clinician to wonder if that child's sadness about being alone is characterized by Self-deprecating statements of unworthiness (*introjective*) or rather more by powerlessness (*anaclitic*). In the former, the needs could be characterized as "loss of love" needs. In the latter, there are also components of *exousia* and/or *dunamis* needs that could be explored. These needs would then be addressed through interventions focused on restoring self-esteem and repairing the child's sense of Self in relation to Others and the world, using other standard FELT techniques.

The dynamic theories described above are just a small portion of the many ideas that would need to be included to adapt a FELT model to depression. Still, it can be seen even in this example that the basic psychological human needs outlined in FELT can apply to depression as well as anxiety. In other words, the human needs outlined in FELT are considered to be universal human needs, and unresolved tension in those needs can lead to multiple symptomatic outcomes, not just anxiety. Thus, those needs can be used to create intervention plans across multiple types of disorders.

In addition to adapting FELT's etiological model to be more specific to depression, it would be necessary also to revise the thematic coding system used to analyze play in FELT to better suit the play of depressed children. Unfortunately, due to the aforementioned diagnostic rarity of pediatric depression, and the inherent challenges present in identifying purely depressed children (those who have depression, but not anxiety), rigorous, high-quality studies examining the play of depressed children have not emerged at the same level as those that have studied anxiety. The play of anxious children has been heavily studied, using robust methods. The same cannot be said of the play of depressed children. So, a first step in adapting FELT to depressed children would be to better identify and document, using rigorous research methods, how the play of depressed children differs from that of non-depressed children. The narrative coding systems used in the MSSB and in FELT are promising frameworks for starting this work, but likely the most challenging part of conducting such research would be to find enough children who meet criteria for depression to produce good data. Existing studies have not produced consistent, meaningful findings.

To study the play of depressed children, standardized stems that would be expected to elicit potentially meaningful data would need to be created. These would include stories that capture the many scenarios in which depressed affect can emerge, including stories of loss, abandonment, failures, and grief, to name a few. Ideally, these stories would then need to undergo "beta testing" with a relatively small number of children to work out any "kinks" in the stories. Once finalized versions are reached, they could then be implemented in a controlled study with age-matched children with no diagnoses and those with depression. Furthermore, standardized, high-quality methods for identifying children with depression would need to be used to test eligibility for the study. Research assistants would need to be well-trained in clinical interviews with young children and well-trained in the reliable administration of the story stems being studied. As was done with the MSSB, research assistants would also need to first study the stems without applying any intervention. Only after these early studies were completed could we then also develop an intervention plan, and then test the intervention.

Realistically, all these steps are likely to take several years of focused research from teams of researchers. Still, there is great promise in the format proposed within FELT for working in an empirically informed, replicable manner to understand the play of depressed children. From there, interventions could be planned and executed accordingly, focused on addressing core psychodynamic needs through play analysis and integrative play techniques. Furthermore, the example of depression given here is just one example of how the FELT approach could be translated to meet numerous childhood needs.

Notes

1 The symptoms as listed here are paraphrased for readability and brevity.
2 I am using data from 2019 here to help eliminate the well-known effects of COVID-19 on mental health.
3 It should be noted that this assertion primarily pertains to treatment decisions and the surface-level characteristics of effective treatment. There still remain other reasons and contexts in which diagnostic specificity could be quite valuable (see below).

REFERENCES

American Psychiatric Association. (2013). *Diagnostic and Statistical Manual of Mental Disorders* (5th ed.). Washington, DC: American Psychiatric Publishing.

Bibring, E. (1953). The mechanism of depression. In P. Greenacre (Ed.), *Affective Disorders; Psychoanalytic Contributions to Their Study* (pp. 13–48). Madison, CT: International Universities Press.

Daly, M. (2022). Prevalence of depression among adolescents in the U.S. from 2009 to 2019: analysis of trends by sex, race/ethnicity, and income. *Journal of Adolescent Health*, 70(3), 496–499.

Fitzpatrick, O. M., Cho, E., Venturo-Conerly, K. E., Ugueto, A. M., Ng, M. Y., & Weisz, J. R. (2023). Empirically supported principles of change in youth psychotherapy: exploring codability, frequency of use, and meta-analytic findings. *Clinical Psychological Science*, 11(2), 326–344.

Freud, S. (1917). Mourning and melancholia. In J. Strachey (Ed.), *The Standard Edition of the Complete Psychological Works of Sigmund Freud, vol.* XIV *(1914–1916): On the History of the Psycho-Analytic Movement, Papers on Metapsychology, and Other Works* (pp. 243–258). London: The Hogarth Press and the Institute of Psycho-Analysis.

Klein, M. (1940). Mourning and its relation to manic-depressive states. *The International Journal of Psychoanalysis*, 21, 125–153.

Zero to Three. (2016). *DC:0–5 – Diagnostic Classification of Mental Health and Developmental Disorders of Infancy and Early Childhood*. Washington, DC: Zero to Three.

Index

ACER model 92–97
adverse childhood experiences 63, 113
agonists/antagonists 123; inverse agonist, 125
amplifiers 100; situational, 104; stable, 104
anal stage 85
analgesia/comfort needs 104
anxiety: pharmacological approaches to treatment 122; sensitivity 109; temporal factors 98, 111–116, 174
attunement 6, 57, 92–93

Behavioral Approach System 110
Behavioral Inhibition System 110
benzodiazepine 122, 125–127

castration anxiety 101
concern (therapeutic) 94
conservation 64
contextual psychotherapy 14, 95
corrective emotional experience 76, 88, 92
cortisol see HPA
corticotropin-releasing factor see HPA

danger (as a play theme) **17**, 28, 156, 175, 185
depression: anaclitic, 237; introjective, 238
deus ex machina resolution **17**, 21, 176, 183
disintegration anxiety 84, 101–103, 175
distal influences 73, 220

emotional shift **17**, 23, 29, 153, 156, 174
emotions circumplex 150
Erikson's psychosocial stages 87
exousia 77, 79, 184, 227–230
expertise 92, 94
expression/catharsis 76, 88, 92

familiarity 8; and relational 220–222, 230
FELT etiological model of anxiety: general overview 98–99
FELT fidelity checklist 15
FELT themes: overview **17**
final content (as a play theme) **17**, 19, 21, 35, 153, 156
fulfillment (as a thereapeutic need) 123–124, 131

GABA – gamma-amino-butyric acid 125–126, 129
gene by environment (GxE) interactions 100
genital stage 86
good enough objects 56, 57, 66–69, 177

HPA/hypothalamic-pituitary-adrenal axis 128
hydroxyzine 125

incongruent affect **17**, 24–26, 153
initial response **17**, 18, 22, 25, 155, 157
integration: needs, 77, 83–84, 86; object 62, 67; self 102, 175
interoception, 164
interoceptive exposure 132, 164–166; activities for children **165–166**

labeling of emotions and symptoms **17**, 29, 31, 76, 93, 156
latency stage 86
learned helplessness 45

MacArthur Story Stem Battery (MSSB) 16–18
monoamine oxidase (MAO) 124, 130

multilayered stories 227
myelination 114

need for love 77, 80
need for objects 77, 81
neediness (as play theme) **17**, 29–30, 156
negative affect 35, 98, 108, 124, 133, 236
norepinephrine: delivery and transport of, 124; serotonin-norepinephrine reuptake inhibitors, 123; system, 129–130
normal narcissism 25, 43–44, 51, 234, 237
normal symbiosis 63, 81

object constancy 64
object differentiation 58–61
object integration 61–68
objects as internal representations, 33, 56, 64, 71
oral stage 85

persecutory anxiety 102; *see also* popularity needs
persistent anxious cognitions 147
phallic stage 86
play: features 11
play therapy: features 6
popularity needs 77, 82, 176, 213, 216
premature termination 203
prime maladaptive themes 34
progressive muscle relaxation 132, 170
proximal influences 73
psychodynamic needs: seven primary, 77

reactions to inescapable fear/anxiety **17**, 27
responsivity 95

sedation/de-arousal: as therapeutic goal 125, 131, 168, 237
self, development of, 39
self, developmental norms and abnormalities, 51–54
self, distortions 72
self, empty 43
self, false 40, 47
self, protean 42–43
self, saturated 42
self, unified 42, 77, 102
self-efficacy 111, 156, 169; therapeutic activity for, 186
self-representations **17**, 31, 43, 46, 49, 72, 156
separation-individuation 63–64, 228
serotonin: behavioral improvement of 133–134; modulation by norepinephrine 129; selective serotonin reuptake inhibitor (SSRI) 123, 130; serotonin-norephinephrine reuptake inhibitor (SNRI) 123; synthesis by tryptophan 134; transport and delivery of 124
split archetypes 66–67
splitting 57, 60–65
storytelling 7–9, 28, 29; as relaxation method 163
superego anxiety 134
superego needs 77, 79, 102, 225
suppressors 100, 116, 131, 137; situational, 103; stable, 103

temporal factors 111–116
therapeutic play 6
tripartite model of anxiety and depression 108

For Product Safety Concerns and Information please contact our EU representative GPSR@taylorandfrancis.com Taylor & Francis Verlag GmbH, Kaufingerstraße 24, 80331 München, Germany

Printed and bound by CPI Group (UK) Ltd, Croydon, CR0 4YY

08/06/2025

01897006-0011